The
East/
Exercise

The East/West Exercise Book

David Smith

McGraw-Hill Book Company

New York
St. Louis
San Francisco
Düsseldorf
Mexico
Toronto

23456789RABP79876

Library of Congress Cataloging in Publication Data
Smith, David Miln.
    The east/west exercise book.
    Bibliography: p.
    1. Exercise. 2. Hygiene. I. Title.
RA781.S59   613.7'1   75-43804
ISBN 0-07-058985-2
ISBN 0-07-058986-0 pbk.

Photographs in this book by Lee Marshall.
Illustrations copyright © 1976 by Claudia Porges.

Dedicated

to

raising

the

health

of

EVERYBODY

Becky,

I thought that this would be an ideal gift for you because of the subject, the dedication, and the fact that you know the author personally! All my love + kisses and Merry Christmas!

I love you,

Stephanie
Christmas '76'

I affectionately and respectfully
acknowledge the teachers from
whom I have derived much
benefit:

Yogi Bhajan,
Paul Curtis,
Oscar Ichazo,
Krishnamurti,
Da Liu,
Baba Ramdas,
Warren Robertson,
Sri John Roger,
Swami Satchidananda,
Dr. Seymour P. Smith,
James Wing Woo,
and the many other teachers
throughout the world.

And great thanks to those
who helped put this book together:

David Brink,
Bruce Comer,
Danny Fields,
Rebecca Ingalls-Smith,
and Karen Williams.

Part Four

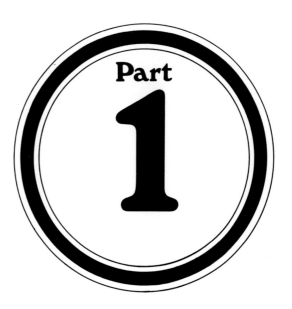

Part

1

Chapter
1

What This Book Can Do for You

How do you feel? Does your body move as easily and freely as you would like it to?

Are you facing a crisis of well being? Are you frequently tired? Do you feel out of shape—and look it? Are you forever thinking about what you should do but not doing it? Do you think of exercise as something you'll get to later, something you're too busy for this week? When will "later" be? It might be too late.

Be honest with yourself; rationalizing drains your energy and avoids facing the truth. Exercise, on the other hand, restores and creates energy. Don't you need more energy—and isn't that why you picked up this book?

People are usually motivated by what they need, and most of us could change our habits if we really wanted to. Don't wait. Let this book work for you now. You have the potential to develop and maintain health and well being right now.

This book contains a unique and complete exercise program, made up from a wide variety of disciplines: ancient and modern, Oriental, European, and American. And, this book is aimed at a wide variety of people—people of all ages, people of both sexes, people with all types of previous training, or none at all. Middle-aged people, students, athletes in their prime, and children have all used, and benefited from, the E/W program.

Results are both immediate and long-range. After the first simple stretching and bending exercises, you will feel more supple, and you will actually *be* more graceful. In a very short while, you will surpass what you once thought of as your limits. Over a longer period, your body will become stronger, more flexible, more vigorous. Your endurance will increase tremendously: activities that now leave you aching and breathless will become virtually effortless. Your circulation will improve, and with it your hair and skin. You will look and feel better than you do today. All you have to do now is begin.

Most likely you've tried exercise books and programs before—and quit. Did you once pick up an intriguing book of yoga exercises, only to find you were so discouragingly far from being able to duplicate all those fascinating positions that you were instantly turned off? Did you then try one of those 10-minute-a-day programs, which required ever-increasing numbers of calisthenic-type exercises? And did you then do them for a couple of weeks or months, until you were thoroughly bored and it became a chore to do them everyday?

We know that most people have started some sort of exercise program and have been unable (or unwilling) to continue. That is why *The East/West Exercise Book* uses a completely different approach.

In the very beginning you are asked not to do the exercises, but to merely visualize yourself doing them. It has been known in the East, and it is now generally accepted in the West, that thought is a form of energy. Merely visualizing yourself doing the exercises will start subtle changes. The E/W exercises have been laid out in a set of cycles which become progressively more difficult, yet are easily learned. By the time you finish one series you are ready for the next. The exercises help relax key pockets of tension, they also help develop balance, flexibility, coordination, strength, and endurance. When you reach the top of the last series you will be able to add to or develop a program suited to your unique individual needs.

Correct breathing, which is overlooked in most programs, is essential in the E/W exercises. You will learn breathing techniques that can be used in your daily activities. Relaxation, so important to the vital and active person, is an integral part of the exercises. The awareness of grounding (the experience of being connected to the earth) and centering (focus of awareness below the navel), formerly unknown in Western exercises, is a feature of the E/W program.

One of the main reasons the E/W exercise program is different from other exercise programs is that it combines different types of exercises. It is based on my experience that for most people no one type of exercise fills all our needs.

Body building, weight training, isometrics, and isotonics produce muscles, tone, and sometimes strength, but rarely do they produce flexibility or endurance. Hatha yoga is well rounded, promoting flexibility, balance, and stimulation of internal organs and glands—but without spending much time practicing advanced postures and breathing techniques, there is little strength or endurance. Endurance training produces strength, stamina, and grounding but little for specific internal stimulation and flexibility. T'ai Chi, Kung Fu and mime help develop grounding, centering, flexibility, balance, and coordination, but do little for endurance. But when you combine and complement these different exercises and approaches—as is done in this book—you have a well-rounded fitness program. The East/West exercise program is designed to help you in every area: strength, stamina, coordination, flexibility, balance, relaxation, breathing, grounding, centering, and health.

Most of the E/W exercises have been around for thousands of years. They come from Hatha yoga (path of physical health); Kundalini yoga (movement of spinal energy); Kung Fu (Chinese path of physical exercise and self-defense—"hard" form); T'ai Chi (Chinese path of physical exercise and self-defense—"soft" form); Arica (Western physical training based on Eastern disciplines); bioenergetic exercise (based on a Western psychoanalytical approach to the expression of feeling); endurance training (develops heart, lungs, and stamina); mime (performing art without the use of words); and isometrics and isotonics (muscular contraction using force against a stationary object and exercising the muscles over their full range of motion, respectively).

The book is organized to help you learn about the different types of exercises and disciplines, their background, and how they can help you. After beginning the exercise program, there is a section on how you can easily integrate exercise into your round of daily activities, at the office or school. The "Games to Freedom" section discusses a change in attitude toward sports, games, and your body. Our discussion of games suggests different ways of channeling your newly created energy into fun and pleasure while developing self-awareness and the attributes of a healthy being. "Other Ways of Healing" emphasizes the need for understanding how to prevent body weakness and the susceptibility to illness to which it leads. The section on nutrition teaches the simple principles of which you should be aware. "Help for Special Problems" is a cross-reference index provided so that you can easily find exercises to help any problems in specific areas. Finally, "Concentration/Meditation" gives you several simple techniques and ideas on meditation.

The East/West Exercise Book is a book of action. It works only if you work with it. Some of the ideas and actions may seem alien to you at this time. That's okay; leave the idea for now with an open mind—and reconsider it in the future.

Chapter 2

A Healthy Body Moves Free and Easy

A healthy body moves free and easy. It is unencumbered by aches and pains, the dead weight of sluggish organs and tensed muscles. It is light and ready to move, from the moment it opens eagerly to the day, until its comfortable folding down for the night. Perfect health is the birthright of every body. The unity of the healthy body and its parts and functions all cooperate for the achievement of the maintenance and perfection of life.

A healthy body sustains a healthy intellect with zest, energy, enthusiasm, vigor, and courage. The personality we manifest and the way we feel about ourselves are directly related to the freedom the body is given in expressing itself. Through movement a person reveals much of his inner life. A healthy body animates the enjoyment of life.

Growing up need not mean you can no longer expect to "sleep like a baby" or wake up zestfully with a hearty appetite for living. Watch a baby. A healthy infant is a study in motion. Head, arms, legs, lungs, torso—every nerve and muscle vibrates, alternatively pushing out and pulling in, throbbing between tension and release, uninhibited, instinctive and free. These seemingly spasmodic actions express a perfectly coordinated system in which each part is interrelated and interacting. A healthy body is one in which organs, nerves, and muscles cooperate to maintain a symmetry of body rhythms.

None of the suppleness, enthusiasm, or amazing endurance of a baby (it can body-cry for hours without exhaustion) need be lost in adulthood. There are outlets for body motion which should be utilized if you hope to sustain your original gift of health. You cannot stop moving (exercising) or breathe incorrectly and still expect to have a baby's powerful lungs, vibrant diaphragm, elastic intestines, and strong heart. Nor will your nerves be steady enough or your mind clear enough to handle the mental and emotional challenges of adulthood.

Moving through the day with a natural charge of energy, without false stimulation from caffeine, nicotine, or pep pills, is the inherent right of everyone. The type of exhilaration that emanates from a baby should be the native state of a healthy body, regardless of age. Adult good health is a sophisticated version of an infant's agility, charm, and even muscular strength (which is relative, of course, but try pulling your finger away from a baby's grasp). These are not toys to be put away when you grow up—they are gifts inherited for life and, without them, health breaks down.

Internal cleanliness, relaxed and sturdy inner organs working cooperatively together, are the best prevention against disease. A healthy body can tolerate foreign bacteria without breaking down.

The unhealthy body frequently reacts improperly to stress, a stimulus to the emotions that provokes the body to react. Failure to release the body responses generated by stress can cause inhibition—centers of tension resulting in colitis, high blood pressure, nervousness, headaches, ulcers, heart disease, emotional insecurity, and many other ills. Dr. Hans Kraus, an internationally known back specialist, says, " . . . tension, or lack of flexibility, is responsible for more attacks of back pain than any other single cause."

To understand why this happens we must understand the ancient principle of "fight or flight." Whatever personal or social restraints we may inflict upon ourselves in response to anger, anxiety, fear, or daily minor and major irritations, our body interprets this age-old message as a biological need for sudden spurts of adrenalin and blood and for tensed muscles—in short, the body must be ready for action.

When no action occurs, when we want to stamp in anger or jump in joy, we freeze or tighten up. The biological responses of our bodies begin to work against us, blood pressure builds, muscles become snagged in tension, and internal juices start consuming devitalized organ tissue. Sooner or later a symptom of disease develops. You go to the doctor and the symptom is treated and (you hope) eliminated. But, unless you deal with stress and tension, you will be back in the doctor's office with the same or a different ill.

Three world-renowned specialists, Dr. Paul Dudley White, the heart specialist, Dr. Hans Selye, and Dr. Hans Kraus, both authorities on the subject of stress, all concur that "lack of exercise combined with constant irritation produces an imbalance, a sickness in our emotional and physical functions." We are bombarded with different types of stress daily. City dwellers are constantly hit with noise from cars and industry, pollution from water and air. Unless we are careful, much of our food will be loaded with poisons. There is physical and mental stress from overwork producing fatigue and perhaps later disease.

But there are positive aspects of stress. Stress in sports, games, arts, crafts, music, and accomplishment represents a challenge to the human organism, an opportunity to test one's strength and become stronger physically, mentally, and spiritually. As such, it is a healthful part of being alive. The E/W exercise program, though a stressor itself, can eliminate the negative effects of many tension sources by serving as an outlet, by strengthening the body and progressively adapting it to a greater level of health.

When stress is internalized and not transformed into a form of action or productivity/creativity, the energy flow shuts down. Stress, having no outlet, begins to prey on the body and the mind.

Restoring the body to a healthful level of activity in our society requires the constructive use of tension and stress to buttress the body—to release a positive flow of energy. The achievement of good health needs a certain degree of physical and psychological stress to convert the pressure of daily living into the positive stress of exercise.

The physical activity of E/W exercise works best against mental and emotional stress. The relaxation techniques are most effective in easing physical stress. You will be more aware of your energy and be able to direct it for your—and everyone else's—good.

Chapter 3

The Best of East and West

Traditionally, Western man has placed great emphasis on reason and progress, whereas Eastern man has emphasized the values of trust, faith, service, and love. To the Western man, the mind has been regarded as an ally in the struggle against nature; the Eastern man has seen the mind as his enemy and nature as his ally. But today we are witnessing a remarkable phenomenon—the West is becoming Easternized, and the East is becoming Westernized. A synthesis is taking place, to the benefit of both civilizations. No longer do reason and progress alone hold exclusive dominion over the civilization of the West. The time is come when other values and other ways of looking at man and the human condition are being given their due.

From this blending of civilizations has come the East/West exercise program. Until now, most exercise programs have not given the human being a total balance. But, as we have said, E/W is an eclectic system, taken from many of the world's old and new disciplines. These disciplines have been combined to form an easily learned program which can be modified to suit your individual needs.

Of course, you will find adherents of particular systems who will tell you that theirs is the only way. Years of teaching and studying the various disciplines have indicated to us that—for the great majority of people—there is no single way that takes care of all of a person's needs. You can love and learn from them all.

For that reason, we have set out to develop a system that incorporates the most effective principles, procedures, and goals of many different systems. The E/W system is the result of extensive experimentation and research. It is a flexible system that benefits the entire body, and it is particularly suited to the requirements of men and women living in Western societies, where time (and patience) are likely to be limited.

If you have specific health problems, you should, of course, consult a physician before engaging in E/W exercises.

The following is a brief background of each of the disciplines used in E/W. After having read through each, you should be familiar and comfortable enough with them to begin doing the exercises themselves.

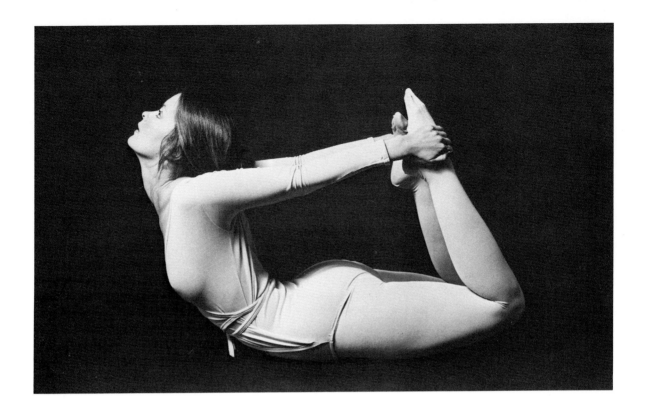

Yoga

Yoga is the science of spiritual self-development that has been taught in India for thousands of years. The Sanskrit word *yoga* means "union"—of mind, body, and spirit of the Individual Self with the Infinite Self.

There are several main paths of yoga. Hatha yoga, (*ha* = sun, *tha* = moon), the path of physical health, is the one with which we are primarily concerned.

Yogis, or those who practice yoga, say that purity of the mind is not possible without purity of the physical body. Purity of the body is attained through the use of postures (asanas), breath control (pranayama), cleansing processes (kriyas) and deep relaxation, all of which are incorporated in E/W exercises.

Yoga postures in this book have been scientifically worked out to put the right amount of pressure on organs and glands to stimulate, massage and balance them. The head stand and shoulder stand, for instance, allow the organs to be stimulated by moving upside-down from their routine position. In the shoulder stand, with the chin tucked into the neck, the angle and position of the body create pressure on the thyroid and parathyroid glands in the neck. The shoulder and head stands also help venous bloodflow and thus relieve leg tension and varicose veins.

Breath control, pranayama, is an important part of yogic discipline. Better breathing technique means more air intake. More air is more oxygen—and more oxygen, in turn, means increased endurance and vitality. Ancient spiritual texts and contemporary yogis claim that a vital energy substance called "prana" is responsible for all life activity. Prana is defined as "essential vital force." The utilizing of this prana is what maintains the life of the body.

An advanced use of breathing involves rhythmic inhalation coupled with an active willing of the prana to a specific place for healing, stimulation of a sluggish organ, or a general increase in vitality.

Hatha yoga techniques will promote internal balance, stimulating organs and glands by putting the body into the correct postures. This is an experience that most other exercise techniques do not effect. The yoga techniques will help you become more flexible by stretching the tension out of muscles. Relaxation is one of the prime benefits derived from Hatha yoga as a result of the breathing and stretching techniques Hatha stresses. These techniques are combined in the E/W program to stimulate a high level of health.

Westerners have previously thought their organs functioned involuntarily. Now, however, Western scientific research machines have proven the Hatha yogi to have control over the autonomic nervous system and internal organs. Yoga hospitals in India are curing heart trouble, diabetes, kidney disease, glandular disorders, asthma, blood pressure, arthritis, etc. The list is long. The only requirement is that the patient must be able to get out of bed to do the postures, breathing, and cleansing. E/W employs many of these methods—including a special section on cleansing, so that you can use some of the yogis' techniques for improved hygiene.

14

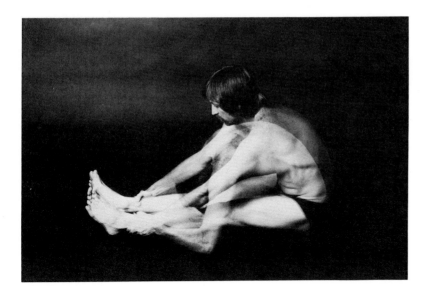

Kundalini Yoga

Kundalini is the name given in ancient Hindu texts to a very subtle form of biological energy which lies dormant (in most people) at the base of the spine between the anus and the genitals. The release of this energy is said to be intimately involved in the development of higher consciousness. The concept of Kundalini is not limited to Hindu teaching alone. It has been described in the ancient esoteric literatures of China, Egypt, Sumer, and Greece, among others.

In the Hindu tradition, Kundalini means "coiled serpent." It implies latent energy. Kundalini is symbolized as a sleeping serpent coiled three and a half times around the base of the spine at the point called the Root or Basic Chakra. Chakra is a Sanskrit term meaning "wheel," "energy vortex," or "spiritual center." There are seven of these centers. Western science identifies the site of the seven spiritual centers as the locations of seven endocrine glands and six nerve plexuses.

Each of these centers is the focus for a set of basic attitudes about life that determines our behavior. Our behavior, in turn, influences these centers. Each center needs to be balanced within itself and with every other center. When this has progressed to a certain stage, the Kundalini will start to rise. A center becomes more balanced as the attitudes of the person relating to that center become more real—that is, harmonious with the laws of Life.

When Kundalini awakens it travels up the spinal cord through the path made clear by the balancing and opening of the six spiritual centers and connects like an electric charge (planetary lightning) with the Crown (or seventh) Chakra. He who experiences this phenomenon attains the ultimate superconscious state—Supreme Knowledge.

The Kundalini itself and the process of awakening are very mysterious. Many people have awakened a small amount of this energy and don't know it. It has imperceptibly filtered into their normal energy life. Those in whom this has occurred are most gifted. Kundalini is a creative energy. It is said that the inspiration and intuition of the artist and scientist are propelled and sustained by this energy and that a person's sense of meaning and enthusiasm for life also depend on it.

The body is the physical bearer of Kundalini energy. The stronger and cleaner the body is, the more current it can carry safely. E/W focuses on the physical aspects of the development of consciousness. The other important areas of development can be found elsewhere.

The Kundalini postures used in E/W were introduced to America by Yogi Bhajan from India. According to Yogi Bhajan, "A healthy person is one who has no disease. . . . A happy person is one whose mind is clear. He can become his own source of inspiration for those who are falling apart around him."

Arica

Arica Institute, which has centers throughout the United States, teaches an intensive training in conscious evolution, a method for developing a person's consciousness so that higher states of awareness become permanently available.

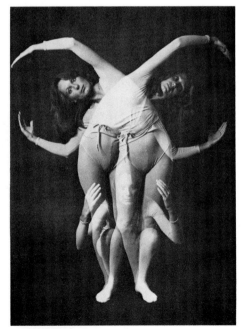

Arica, like E/W, considers that man is born essential, natural, and spontaneous and, as a natural process of learning, is conditioned by his society, parents, teachers, and religion into fixed patterns of perception and behavior. The science of Arica involves a method for processing this conditioning so that man can regain his essential self. He once again has the freedom of a baby, but he retains all the useful knowledge he has absorbed from his culture while growing up.

Bioenergetic Exercise

Bioenergetics was developed by Dr. Alexander Lowen and Dr. John Pierrakos of New York from the work begun by Wilhelm Reich. It is a psychiatric discipline that uses analysis of body structure as its primary therapeutic tool. Those who practice bioenergetics work from the conviction that the body is an accurate outside picture of the inner life of the individual. The body never lies—it is a precise gauge of a person's psychic state.

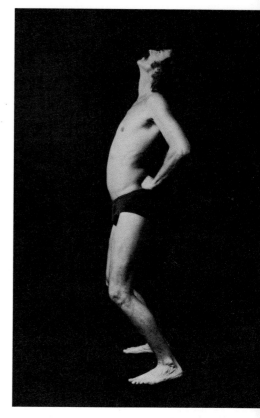

The diagnosis phase of the therapy has two aspects. First, by looking at the body and any limitation of body motility, it can be seen where emotional trauma has distorted the natural perfection of the body line. While distortion can be caused by a flaccid, flabby body it can also be caused by the overtensing of muscles. Initially this tensing was done semiconsciously in order to "stop painful feelings" that had been aroused during an event early in the person's life. If the person was unable to deal satisfactorily with the terms of the early situation, they remain still vulnerable to these painful feelings and so must maintain the tense muscles as a defense—and thus there is a loss of awareness in the muscles.

The second aspect of this diagnosis concerns the exact location and effect of this tension. This information reveals important facts about the person's inner life and hence the source of distress which the therapist works with.

Bioenergetics recognizes the importance of full deep breathing. It is the therapists' experience that tension anywhere in the body restricts breathing. Different aspects of breathing are explored in this therapy, particularly the propensity to stop breathing under stress. Bioenergetics says, "The inability to breathe freely under emotional stress is the physiological basis for the experience of anxiety in such stressful situations." E/W incorporates bioenergetic exercises to develop a bodymind that moves and breathes in stress and play.

The areas of tense muscles are referred to as "blocks." This word is chosen because tense muscles block the natural flow of energy through the body. Too, a healthy relaxed muscle experiences no pain under reasonable pressure. These blocks must be dissolved. This is accomplished in two ways. The first is with continuous direct pressure, as in massage. The second is with exercise. Many of the exercises deliberately put the body in a position of stress and vulnerability. The stress makes it more difficult for the muscles to "keep the feeling trapped." Through the right psychoanalytical approach—along with skillfully applied pressure—the muscles can release, and the person, when ready, finally can express the feeling. The expression of feeling releases energy, which then circulates through the body. This starts the body healing itself; the person feels an increase in vitality, alertness, and freedom. We only have one feeling track and therefore, insofar as we restrict so-called "bad" feelings, we also restrict our capacity to experience "good" feelings. As we confront, make conscious, and release painful feelings, our capacity to feel well also increases.

Grounding is another area that gets considerable attention in bioenergetic exercise. As more and more energy is released in the body, it is necessary to anchor it, to utilize it in the person's outer world. This is aided through grounding. Relaxing into the earth and experiencing its support encourages us to invest our energy and create, here and now, whatever creativity has given our hands and hearts and minds to do.

Kung Fu

Kung Fu is a generic term that means "discipline" or "exercise." It includes both the physical training of a martial art and the physical training for health. Properly, the martial art is called Wu-shu. Wu-shu was the original impetus for the development of the exercises for health. The common people, impressed by the physical prowess of the Kung Fu men of their time, started doing the exercise themselves out of concern for

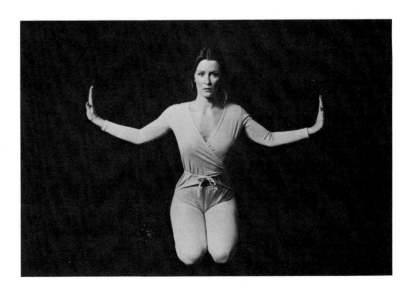

their personal health. This initial development took place sometime prior to 2674 B.C.

The life and work of Lao-tse, and the subsequent development of Taoism, had an important effect on Kung Fu. It provided the art with a philosophy to stimulate and guide its further development. Breathing techniques, meditation, medicine, and alchemy became part of the Kung Fu man's equipment.

Through the many years that followed, the arts split into many styles. The two main lines were described as the Hard School and the Soft School. The former developed power, strength, and aggression. The latter developed slowness, softness, and calm; it became known as T'ai-Chi Chuan—an art which, used by a master, can "defeat a thousand pounds with a force of four ounces."

T'ai Chi

T'ai Chi is a physical culture/martial art. The name means "supreme ultimate." The Chinese consider it one of the pathways to the self. It has been referred to as "metaphysical boxing."

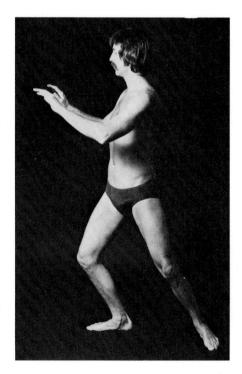

T'ai Chi's grace and slowness of pace make it as beautiful to watch as it feels to do. Arms and legs, head and torso move effortlessly together in balance, lightness, calm, and focus, with legs and feet securely grounded.

The literal action of T'ai Chi—that part of the art that can be seen from the outside—consists of a series of movements that articulate thirty-nine postures. The movements are done very slowly, as though they were being performed under water. It is suggested that one be involved in the movements and not be distracted by any extraneous thoughts that may occur. Thus, for the practice time anyway, one is a single organic unit living in the present time alone.

T'ai Chi develops and instills a number of important elements simultaneously: relaxation, grounding, balance, coordination, strength, and suppleness. It is a very efficient form of exercise.

The first, and for a long time the most important, consideration is relaxation. Nothing of value can happen without it. T'ai Chi requires that one "let go of the body" entirely. Here he who yields learns to overcome he who is strong. To let go seems disorienting—like being set adrift in space—yet the instruction is very clear and allows no exceptions. The body must be absolutely open and "soft" to allow for the development and flow of chi.

Chi is the material of "essential vital force." Indian yoga refers to it as "prana." But, where the yogi says that prana is in the air and enters the bloodstream through the lungs, the Chinese say that chi generates in the area below the navel. This area is referred to as the *tan t'ien*, meaning the "field of seeds." The Chi, then, is said to condense in the bones and eventually permeate the whole body, bestowing ultimate health and vitality on the deserving practitioner. Extreme longevity has been noted in a number of highly accomplished T'ai Chi masters. E/W utilizes many of the basic principles of T'ai Chi.

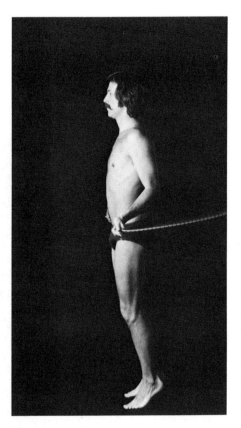

Endurance Training

Endurance training or aerobic exercise is strenuous and sustained just long enough to demand oxygen without causing a craving or an oxygen debt. A strong, balanced, agile, relaxed body means little if it cannot sustain an activity for a prolonged period without fatigue. One method of endurance conditioning is oxygen consumption through physical exercise of the large skeletal muscles, moving the entire body—for example, through running, running in place, swimming, cycling, and rope jumping. E/W incorporates exercises that produce a sustained heart rate of at least 150 beats per minute (after progressive buildup). This naturally forces the lungs to breathe and consume more oxygen than normal. The body's need for oxygen is directly proportionate to its amount of activity. The more active the body, the greater its need. To meet the increased energy expenditure, the oxygen requirement is instantaneously increased to a new level.

The effect of the increased heartbeat and intake of oxygen during exercise in a progressive program increases the efficiency of the cardiovascular and respiratory systems. The resting heart now has a decrease in beats per minute, but an increase in the amount of blood pumped per stroke. The heart gets more rest as it becomes stronger. The body adjusts more quickly to stress and can handle more stress. Because more oxygen is getting to the muscle tissue, the removal of lactic acid is more efficient, thus reducing and delaying fatigue. All the beneficial effects of proper breathing are strengthened and insured with endurance exercise. E/W incorporates several endurance training exercises: running in place, body swings, jumping rope. "For producing the greatest fitness in the least amount of time, nothing surpasses the simple jump rope," according to Dr. Kaare Rodahl, head of the Institute of Work Physiology in Oslo, Norway. There is no question that jumping rope improves cardiovascular efficiency, balance, and coordination. For cardiovascular efficiency, 10 minutes of rope jumping is equal to 30 minutes of jogging.

Exercise enthusiasts have claimed for years that physical activity can improve one's outlook and make one more at ease, more graceful, and more relaxed. A recent study conducted by A. H. Ismail and Robert Young in the Purdue physical education department showed the effects of endurance experience on the personalities of sixty middle-aged men. These men were largely unfit—by any physical fitness standards. Most led sedentary lives as professors and administrators of the university. The group trained for one and a half hours three times a week for four months. Most of the program was progressive supervised running. When the experiment began, few could run more than a quarter of a mile. By the time it ended, they were averaging two to three miles. The main psychological benefit acquired was an increased independence and sense of control over their own life. In addition, their imaginations were said to have increased markedly.

Mime

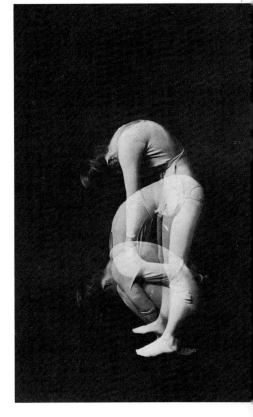

Mime is an ancient performing art dating back to the Egyptian theater. Throughout the East, from India to China, it remains the basic performing element of all theater forms to this day. In the West, there has been a direct historic and geographic progression of mime schools from Egypt through Greece to Rome, where mime was the major theater form for a thousand years, to Italy, France and now the United States.

The most advanced form of this art today is seen in the work of the American Mime Theater. Paul J. Curtis founded this theater in New York in 1952.

Curtis, attempting to put together a theater company, found that actors couldn't move and dancers couldn't act. Since that time he has worked continuously to develop the American Mime Theater as a medium to combat those problems. The physical technique of the Mime Theater develops strength and control. It also develops spontaneity and a greatly expanded imagination and ability in the use of the body. The students learn to think and express themselves symbolically and to create their own mime plays. E/W uses some of these techniques in the cycles and in the "Games to Freedom." For the student, the techniques help to remove the limitations of conventional social experience to produce a creative state and the ability to move and act simultaneously. Dropping inhibitions which may be defined as inner impediments to free expression leads to a positive spirited enjoyment of life.

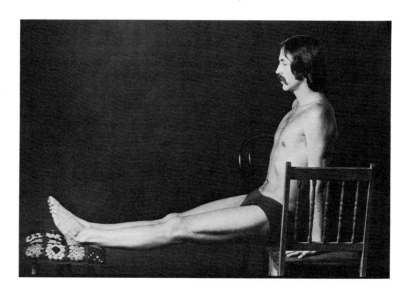

Isometrics/Isotonics

An isometric exercise, more commonly known as an exercise in dynamic tension, is a muscular contraction in which you exert force against a resistance that does not move—either another set of your own muscles or a stationary object. We've all played the game of standing in a doorway pushing the back of our wrists against the door frame; that's an isometric. *Iso* means "equal"; *metric*, "measure." Isometrics helps to strengthen and tone muscles, and E/W includes isometric techniques (for example, hand presses to lift and give life to sagging chests).

Isotonic exercises are the opposite of isometrics in that they produce movement. They exercise the muscles over their full range of motion, which is important in maintaining flexibility. Weight-lifting and calisthenics fall into this type. Isotonic exercise promotes muscle strength if done with the right amount of progression, repetition, and weight or pressure. Too often, however, this type of activity is engaged in to the exclusion of other important inner requirements of the body. However, as a supplement to other exercises, isotonics has a positive overall effect.

Isotonics can be used to develop strength for a particular movement. A batter or a golfer can position his body and a heavier than normal club or pipe in a manner that will simulate contact with the ball, like a practice swing. Muscles used in the swing will develop by exerting the body maximally in that position. E/W uses this technique in "Games to Freedom."

Heart-Rate Monitoring for Endurance Training

Periodic monitoring of your heart rate—your pulse—helps maximize your involvement in the endurance training exercises. Knowing your heart rate tells you whether to increase or decrease the pace at which you are running or jumping rope so you can gradually build endurance.

The dynamics of the exercise plays an important part in the response of the heart rate, although other factors also affect the rate—i.e., time of day, food intake, amount of sleep, and emotional state (particularly in a competitive event).

In E/W you are concerned with three types of exercises with variations (jumping rope, running in place, body swings) that will raise your heart rate enough to cause cardiovascular and respiratory endurance.

If, for example, you do the jump rope exercise in the first chart, after 50 steps you may monitor your heart rate at 90 beats per minute. After looking at the heart-rate schedule for your age, you may discover you must increase your pace. While running in place, if you feel dizzy and breathless, you should stop immediately. If you are curious and you check you pulse, the rate may measure 185! These three indications—dizziness, breathlessness, and high pulse rate—tell you to slow down your pace. You have plenty of time; it's a long-range program.

Age	Heart Rate				
Cycle	I	II	III	IV	V
16–20	130–140	140–150	150–160	160	165–175
21–25	130–140	140–150	150–160	160	165–175
26–30	125–135	135–145	145–155	155	160–170
31–35	120–130	130–140	140–150	150	155–165
36–40	115–125	125–135	135–145	145	145–155
41–45	110–120	120–130	130–140	140	140–150
46–50	110–120	120–130	130–140	140	140–150
51–55	100–110	110–120	120–130	130	130–140
56–60	100–110	110–120	120–130	130	130–140
61–65	95–105	105–115	115–125	125	125–135
66+	95–105	100–110	110–120	120	120–130

Keep heart rate approximately within suggested boundaries of schedule.

One of the best techniques for taking your pulse is with a hand lightly placed on the throat or chest. Don't press so hard you impede the blood flow. Start counting 5 seconds after you stopped the exercise, counting: zero, one, two, three, etc. (Zero marks the beginning of the timed interval.) Take the count for 15 seconds, multiply by four, and you have your pulse rate per minute.

Step Test

This simple test will tell you in a few minutes the recovery rate of your heart—that is, its capacity to return to normal after doing taxing activity.

All you need to take the test is a watch with a second hand and a sturdy bench or chair which rises 15–17 inches off the ground and you're ready to begin. First, take your heart rate at a resting pace. Sometimes it is hard to find your heartbeat—try your wrist, the artery at side of your throat, or your heart. Remember to count zero on the first beat, then one, two, etc.

Next step up onto the chair, one leg following the other so that your legs are straightened; then step down, with one leg followed by the other. It is a four-count rhythm—up, up, down, down. This counts as one step. You do 30 a minute for 2 minutes, or 60 steps, one every 2 seconds.

The second part of the test is monitoring your heart rate and recovery. To keep the test as accurate as possible start the stepping when the second hand hits 12 o'clock and stop when it hits 2 minutes later—even if you haven't reached 60 steps or if you are well past 60 steps. After doing the test a few times and watching the clock, you will get the right rhythm and time.

Take your heart rate five seconds after you finished stepping (at 1 o'clock) for 15 seconds (multiply by four to get the minute rate). When the second hand hits 1 o'clock again, take your heart rate again for 15 seconds (multiply times 4). This is the important figure—your heart recovery rate. It should be under 100. And it *will* be in a few months with exercise and endurance training. You can continue to take your heart rate for the next few minutes just to see how long it takes your heart to recover fully.

Combined together in the E/W program, the different disciplines described in this chapter complement and reinforce one another. The soft methodical pattern of T'ai Chi flows into the limitless movements of the American mime, creating balance, poise, and grace. The kicks of Kung Fu and dynamic movement of Kundalini yoga complement the grounding process of bioenergetics, reawakening the feet, legs, and pelvic area. Endurance conditioning's continued demand for oxygen works directly on cardiovascular and respiratory endurance, stimulating the heart to beat rapidly, while an Arica exercise helps bring the muscles and breath back to normal. Isotonic pushups for men and lightweight isotonic and isometric exercises for women give strength to arms and shoulders and an aesthetically attractive look to the chest, while Hatha yoga makes the body flexible, supple, and relaxed and stimulates the organs and glands.

E/W brings this eclectic system together. Energize your way through each series, teaching yourself to create and maintain good health. Each E/W exercise is designed to develop as many areas as possible. For instance, there is a series of progressive pushups (isotonics) to develop an awareness of balance (standing on your hands) and to give strength to arms, shoulders, and chest muscles. Many people who have never dreamed of doing a hand stand because it seemed too difficult will now learn it in progressive steps. Doing something difficult is always rewarding.

Chapter 4

Healthy Harmony-Four Techniques

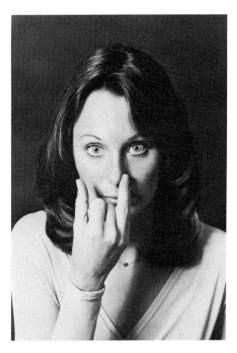

Breathing

Breath is a nectar of life—yet most of us take it for granted. Correct breathing can prolong an energetic life. Restricted shallow breathing—breathing in slow pants—is responsible (except during meditation) for many physical and psychological ills.

Tensions, foul air, and social customs (i.e., keeping a tight tummy) are inhibitions to proper breathing. When happy and relaxed, we breathe freely. When angry, fearful, intimidated, or tense, we freeze up, hold our breath, or pant in rapid rasping gulps. As we free our breath, we relax our emotions and let go of our body tensions.

Proper breathing regulates basic physiological responses. For a body to run efficiently, it must be able to consume a maximum amount of oxygen. If the diaphragm—the flat, sheetlike muscle between the chest cavity and the abdomen—is fully contracted, the lungs can also expand to receive a plentiful supply of air created by the vacuum. As the diaphragm relaxes, the air is expelled.

Tight, shallow breaths do not stimulate the diaphragm into opening up the chest cavity. This muscle, like all others, will atrophy with lack of use, and after years of shallow breathing it becomes inert, while the lungs and chest shrink in and decreasing amounts of air seep through. The body is left ready and waiting for disease.

One of the most damaging habits civilized man has adopted is to breathe in through his mouth. The nose was ingeniously constructed for respiration. It is filled with tiny hairs that filter impurities with mucous membranes to warm the air.

In the East a distinctive element of air is recognized—one that is not recognized in the West. Although it has many names, we'll use the Sanskrit term "prana." As we have said before, prana, to the yogis, is the crucial element within air that kindles vitality and the unique ability to think, exercise free will, and act consciously. This is why a controlled technique of breathing (pranayama), incorporating a maximum intake of air, is an integral part of Eastern exercise. Breathing supplies the oxygen necessary for physical and mental well being.

By breathing in only with the upper portion of the lungs, an inadequate amount of air is circulated. The physical manifestations of this shallow breath are a flattened abdomen and diaphragm, with the collarbone and shoulders hiked up, resulting in minimal breath capacity and an inordinate strain on the body. "Deep diaphragmic or abdominal breathing" is necessary: the diaphragm is activated only by a hearty inhalation that causes the abdomen to pull out, expanding the diaphragm muscle and pushing the lungs open to fill them.

The "yogi complete breath" combines these three motions in one sweeping breath, which starts at the gut level and moves smoothly up through the middle section and finally the upper chest and collarbone. The breath is properly exhaled in the same order after retaining it for a few counts. This method, which can be practiced easily at intervals during the day, provides the greatest physical benefit with the least strain. With each deep breath you inhale a new sense of aliveness, as dulled muscles begin to expand and contract, massaging the internal organs and alerting them to their natural functions.

The combination of a revitalized pure circulation of blood and stimulated organs will restore worn out body systems. As the respiratory system is strengthened, the muscles, organs, and fibers of the digestive and excretory and reproductive systems will be toned and invigorated. Setting aside a few minutes a day to practice the "complete breath" (it can be practiced almost anywhere) and other breathing techniques described in the E/W program will reinforce your program of exercise and relaxation.

Relaxation
Relaxation describes that state in which a muscle and its nerves are temporarily at rest. Nerve activity is electrical in nature and therefore capable of being measured to determine our level of relaxation.

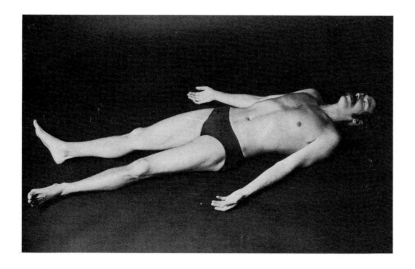

Because we do not live life in a state of total relaxation, we must strive for economy and not waste energy through misdirected nervous activity. In order to know your own appropriate level of nerve activity, you must first learn how to "take all the lines out of the switchboard" and experience total relaxation. Further, in order to rebuild and refresh our bodies during sleep at night, we must learn how to relax both the mind and the body.

The man who originally pioneered basic research in the theory and training of relaxation is Dr. Edmund Jacobson, internist and diagnostician. Dr. Jacobson's approach is to ask the subject to become very quiet, while lying on his back with arms at sides. One muscle is contracted and held, while the subject concentrates on the sensation of tension. When the subject is fully aware of the feeling of tension, the muscle is allowed to go totally limp. The sensation of limpness is contrasted with the previous sensation of tension. In time the subject becomes aware that, while he has created all his tensions, he can dissolve them as well. This approach to relaxation starts an important process that can be described as the development of internal awareness.

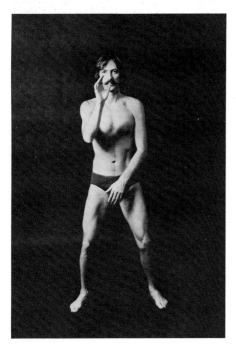

Centering

Centering is a feeling which resembles a "ball of energy" floating below the navel. This center or ball of energy (or gravity) has been placed at spots below the navel or the pit of the stomach.

We develop this center by "circulating awareness" in this area. This is a subtle experience and may not be felt immediately. Give it time. You must remember to relax fully and breathe deeply; relaxing, deep breathing, and centering stimulate balance, creating growth. And you need not restrict this to your exercise periods only; you should practice as often as possible during the day. As you walk, feel the forward motion generating from the lower belly; while running, imagine a line connected from this center to wherever you are running. Let the center carry your body effortlessly through the movement.

Note that centering can refer to the focus of awareness in any center of the body. It is, in short, "the center which directs vital movement and allows us to relate to the world with instinctual immediacy" (Arica).

There are exercises in E/W to help you develop your awareness of this center. Think of it as a soft, warm, light-heavy ball suspended like a gyroscope in the area below your navel. Its position in each of us may vary, but it's about 2–4 inches below the navel in men and slightly lower in women. All movement starts here. The hips swing, legs run and carry the torso, the torso bends and carries the arms from this point.

Grounding

Grounding is the feeling of being connected to, and supported by, the earth. It requires complete confidence in the relationship between your body and what it rests upon.

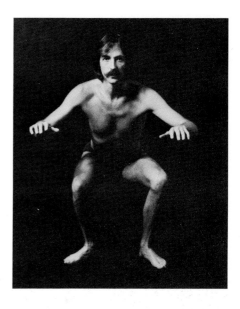

E/W develops grounding by focusing attention on the bottom of the feet, feeling the pressure of contact with the earth, and relaxing the body onto it. Feel the movement in the ankle and make sure it's relaxed; bend the knees and feel as though you are sinking into the earth. Allow the ground to support you.

The most serious obstacle to proper grounding is the habit of locking the knees. When in the locked-knee position, one is standing straight-legged, exerting little or no pressure against the back of the knee. This habit can produce undue strain on the knees and lower back—muscle strain causing leg pain— and can restrict confidence in your ability to hold yourself up. To feel at home in our bodies we need a very real sense of the earth's support.

Breathing, relaxation, centering, and grounding develop slowly. Don't be misled by their apparent simplicity; you will need to practice these exercises patiently. But remember that patience is always important. Without patience we remain mediocre. In E/W you will focus on one aspect at a time until you begin to get a clear sense of each. You can then work on combining them all so that the separate parts merge into one harmonious process. Soon you won't have to think about what you are doing; you will breathe deeply and be relaxed, centered, and grounded in all the activities of your life.

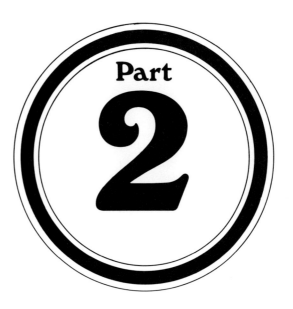

Part

2

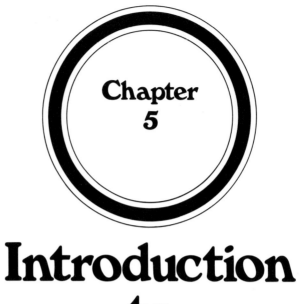

Chapter
5

Introduction to Exercises

E/W exercises are performed in the exact sequence prescribed in each cycle. The cycle is designed to provide a warm-up, slowly increase the heartbeat to a peak, to taper off and relax the body. At the same time it covers key tension pockets, balance, coordination, strength, and endurance. Each cycle prepares you for the next cycle. The number of repetitions and breaths per exercise progresses with your ability to do them correctly. The direction of the program will come from each cycle and you, i.e., what your body can do.

Let me explain. Because we are all in different shape and shapes, each person will respond to the exercises differently and create his or her individual way of handling the amount of repetitions. Since E/W is not one type of exercise, some exercises will be easier than others. The athletic person will easily do the beginning charts of pushups and quickly pick up Kung Fu, but the yoga stretching may be a challenge—and the supple toe-toucher might need endurance training, as well as having to learn the correct way of stimulating the vital organs while stretching.

There is no ladder to climb. For that matter, there will be no need to stop at a certain point because of age or sex. There are some people young in body and mind, yet old in age and knowledge. And, of course, the reverse may be true; young people can suffer from rigid, tense, and aged bodies. E/W will reverse that.

You will start at the minimum number of repetitions in the first cycle. Then you will take from six to eight weeks to get to the maximum number of repetitions in the first cycle. After the first couple of sessions, you will understand the method of the program—and you will have learned much about your body, its strengths and tensions. In a sense, your body will tell you how fast to proceed and how many repetitions to perform.

If you are straining in some or all postures and positions, you should proceed slowly, taking longer than six weeks to reach the maximum number of repetitions in the series. If there are one or two exercises that are particularly difficult, carry them over to the next series or drop them for the present, as you will probably get a variation of them somewhere along the way. It is also a good indication of tension and trouble. If you are moving along smoothly and reach the maximum before six weeks, continue doing the exercise for the six-week period, adding a few repetitions if it feels right.

Each exercise will be introduced by a description of the benefit to be derived from it—that is, the effect the exercise has upon you either immediately or after prolonged use. Next come the instructions on how to execute the exercise, followed by the number of repetitions or the length of time each exercise is performed. The length of time of an exercise is regulated by counting breaths—long/deep or "breath of fire" (short/quick). For example, in Cycle I the forward stretch starts with five long/deep breaths. In Cycle II the forward stretch starts with five long/deep breaths and ends with fifteen breaths of fire.

Do E/W at least four times a week. Don't make excuses to yourself. If your body is very tired one day just do the warm-up—but get to know when you are fooling yourself. If you are, then do the complete series; you will feel better and more energized. Don't rush through the exercises. E/W is flexible enough to be performed for 15 to 40 minutes a day. It's different for everyone. If you have any doubts as to your physical condition in relation to doing E/W exercises, ask your physician.

Since there are many new exercises for the bodymind to learn in Cycle I, you will do eight the first week, ten more the second week, and seven more the third week. By the fourth week you should be totally familiar with Cycle I and doing a total of 25 exercises. This is to insure total comprehension and to give your body time to adjust, adapt, and stretch. After finishing Cycle I you will be comfortable enough with the E/W exercises to do the next cycle in its entirety. Therefore, Cycles II through V will not be divided into smaller groups.

First Week	Second Week	Third Week
(Total exercises: 8)	(Total exercises: 18)	(Total exercises: 25)
Breath of Fire	Breath of Fire	Second week's
Knee Bounce	Knee Bounce	exercises (thru Corpse
Sky/Earth	Sky/Earth	Pose). Add:
Salute to the Sun	Head/Neck Roll	V-Raise No. 1
Corpse Pose	Salute to the Sun	Mule Kick and Arch
Jump Rope or Run in Place	Shoulder Bounce	Scarab
Integration Breath	Pectoral Press	Slow Twist
Contraction/Relaxation	Pushup No. 1	Jump Rope or Run in Place
	Lateral Bend	Knee to Chest
	Situp No. 1	Squat Stand
	Cobra	Shoulder Stand
	Forward Stretch	Fish
	Rock Pose 60°	Contraction/Relaxation
	Camel Ride (Easy Pose)	
	Corpse Pose	
	Jump Rope or Run in Place	
	Integration Breath	
	Contraction/Relaxation	

Before beginning a new cycle, read the exercises and use the photographs as a guide to visualize yourself performing each exercise.

During physical conditioning, the body learns to adjust to the demands placed upon it, in a gradual process of adaptation. As the body masters one level of self-imposed stress in exercise, it readies itself for the next so that, in a sense, a healthy body anticipates challenge and is alert to meet it. Remember that you will be ready to move to the next cycle once you are feeling totally comfortable with the one you are doing. Only a sustained and vigorous program of exercise will energize the heart and flow of blood sufficiently to overcome unexpected stress and ease the normal stress of body activity.

However, even athletes in top condition occasionally experience the side effects of exercise: deep rapid breathing, a pounding pulse and heart, sweating, muscle cramps and soreness, dizziness and fainting. Maintaining the body in sound order minimizes these discomforts and speeds recovery, so that both the process of exercise and its aftermath are more pleasurable.

Nevertheless, muscle cramps and soreness are natural body responses to unfamiliar and intense activity. Cramps are muscle contractions that can be eased by movement or long, hot baths in epsom salts. Soreness may be caused by slight tears in muscle fibers or an accumulation of metabolic wastes. Massage the sore area with a soothing linear heat, and unlike the stiff necks or backaches of emotional tension the discomfort soon will pass.

During exercise, a rapid shift in position may temporarily throw the body off guard, confusing the flow of blood and rhythm of blood pressure. Pressure drops, slowing the delivery of oxygen to the cells, especially to the far corners of the brain. Dizziness and fainting often result, along with cold feet and queasiness as the blood becomes restabilized. Trust your body and let it take charge. Stop the exercise and breathe deeply, and in seconds normal circulation will restore oxygen delivery.

Regular habits of exercise fortify the body for all these experiences. It is generally the weekend athlete who overstrains himself who is susceptible to the dangerous, even fatal, effects of overexercise. The best protection—the best preventative for all disease—is daily, progressive, and habitual healthful conditioning. However, do not hesitate to consult your physician if you feel pain or discomfort.

A positive mental attitude is needed to start E/W exercise. The mental attitude that dictates how inhibited or free our activity will be also controls our response to learning situations. Learning implies stress, because we are exposed to the unknown and therefore we are unsure. If we tighten up, in hostility or in fear, it becomes difficult to learn; all we experience is stress. Mastering a physical skill involves one's state of mind as much as one's motor coordination, balance, or timing.

One more thing: often the concept of competition restrains the individual from learning with paralyzing fears of failure or ridicule. The exercises in this book are for you and you alone, to be followed at your own pace (which will be naturally different from mine or your friend's) for your own goals and with your own needs in mind. These goals and needs cannot possibly be pitted against the goals or needs of anyone else; you are unique and so is your style of learning—and so is what and how you choose to learn.

Get the most you can out of this book. Remember that the book is a map and should not be confused with the truth, which can only be validated by experience. Don't just read it; start the exercises. Learning that which is joyless becomes drudgery. This is for you—enjoy it!

Find a secluded place to do your exercises. A rug with a towel is good; so is a stretch of lawn under a tree. Pick a time of day when you're likely to be bothered the least. The phone disengaged is a good idea. Try different times of the day, then stay with the most comfortable. The morning is the hardest for many people, since their bodies are stiff from sleep—but what a lovely way to begin the day! Some nine-to-fivers prefer exercising after work to relax from the day's tensions and catch a second wind. Whatever time you pick, stick with it.

You'll find some exercises will bring up negativity. If you find this happening, use it. Think of a negative situation that has just happened and that you can't seem to let go of. It may be an "argument" with a total stranger, your boss, or your lover. You keep mulling the confrontation over and what you should have said. If it's unresolved in your mind, substitute the "argument" for the "I-can't-keep-my-legs-up-any-longer"; or do the kicking-out exercises and kick out the "argument." Laugh in the end and you'll probably eliminate the negative thought, liking the person and yourself better for it.

You may enjoy playing these exercise scales on your body instrument with the rhythm and beat of music in the background. The exercises are to have fun with—even when you use them as "negative" exercises that can make you laugh or cry.

Stay in present time with your newly acquired feelings and energy. When in the corpse pose, relax away the past and future films and tapes in your head. Breathe those extraneous things out.

Chapter 6

Cycle I

Warm-Up:

Breath of Fire

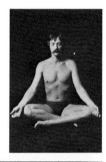

Salute to the Sun

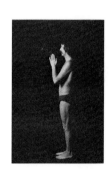

Knee Bounce

Exercises:

Sky/Earth

Shoulder Bounce

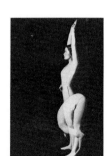

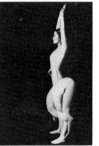

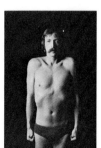

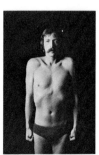

Head/Neck Roll

Pectoral Press

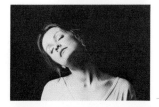

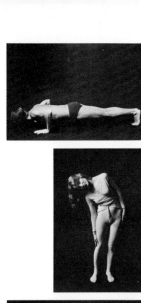
Pushup No. 1

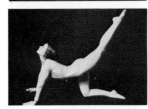
V Raise No. 1

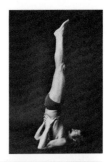
Shoulder Stand

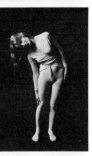
Trunk Lateral Bend

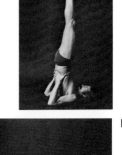
Mule Kick and Arch

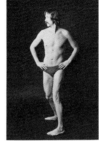
Slow Twist

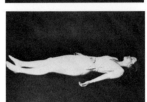
Fish

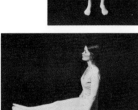
Situp No. 1

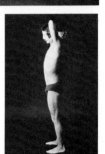
Contraction/ Relaxation

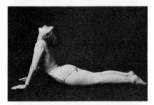
Cobra

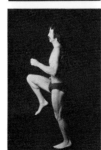
Jump Rope or Run in Place

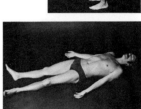
Integration Breath

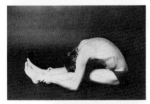
Forward Stretch

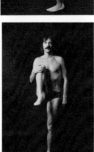
Knee to Chest

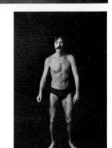
Corpse Pose

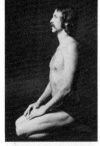
Rock Pose 60°

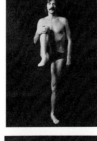
Squat Stand

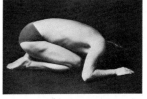
Shake

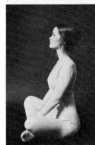
Camel Ride (Easy Pose)

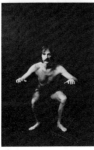
Scarab

Breath of Fire

Stimulates circulation, creates heat, clears head, and restores vitality.

1 Sitting in Easy Pose (sitting on floor, legs crossed in "American Indian style"), forearms over knees, palms up and open, head, neck and trunk in a straight line, inhale through nose into belly.
2 Exhalation is done quickly and forcibly by contracting the abdominal muscles with a backward push.
3 Release abdominal muscles on a short quick inhale through nose.

Do ten breaths of fire; take a long, deep breath and do ten more, then a long, deep breath and ten more, then another deep breath. That's thirty breaths of fire for one round. Do three rounds. If lightheadedness occurs, breathe normally. Place hands just below your navel at first to get the feeling of the diaphragm expanding and contracting. Your abdomen moves forward on the inhalation and flattens on exhalation. A rapid succession of forcible expulsions is the characteristic of the Breath of Fire. The accent is on the exhalation. The Breath of Fire is done sitting, standing, or in any combination of postures.

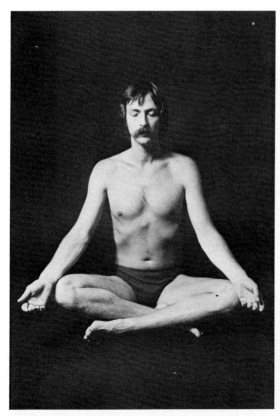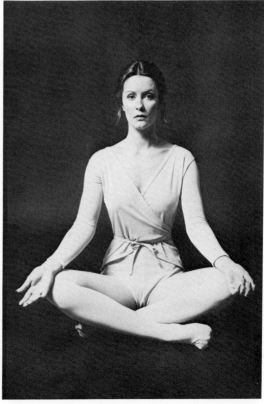

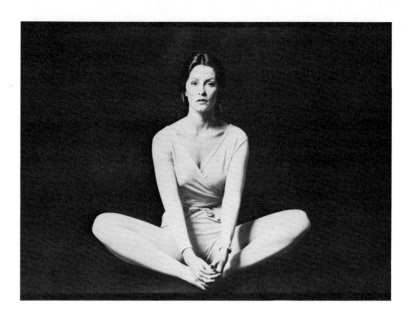

Knee Bounce

This Kundalini knee bounce loosens hip joint and groin tensions and firms and tightens skin and muscles of the inner thighs. It helps in sitting for meditation, too.

1 Sitting on the floor, put the bottom of your feet together.
2 Clasp your fingers together around toes.
3 Bounce knees lightly toward floor.
4 Exhale quickly through nose as knees drop toward floor; inhale as knees are brought up.

It's helpful to close your eyes and mentally say "open up" to the tight groin muscles. Repeat it as you bounce.

Start with twenty breath/bounces; add two per session until you reach fifty.

Sky/Earth

A warm-up stretch taken from Hatha yoga; it starts loosening the neck, shoulder, spine, and legs.

1 Standing, feet at shoulder width and parallel, inhale, raising arms forward and up reaching toward the sky.
2 Exhale and slowly bring arms back to sides. Repeat once.
3 Inhale with arms up, exhale bending from waist; lightly bounce hands and shoulders toward floor three times.
4 Inhale and stretch toward sky; exhale bending from waist.
Repeat sequence twice. Finish with arms at sides.

While bending let go of neck tension, bounce head slightly. Knees can be slightly bent.

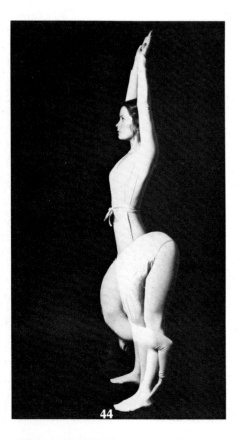

44

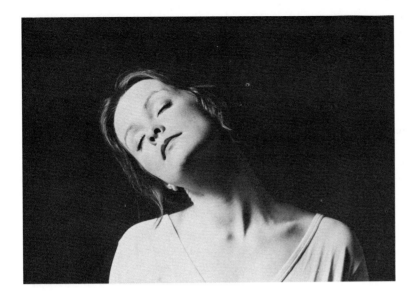

Head/Neck Roll

This Kundalini exercise helps relieve headache and stimulates thyroid gland.

1 Standing, feet inches apart, arms by sides, drop chin to chest.
2 Rub chin lightly on chest side to side; then roll head slowly 360° to the right three times.
3 Change direction and roll head to the left three times.

Relax shoulders, and with eyes closed concentrate on point between eyebrows. Breathe long and deep. Remember to roll slowly.

Salute to the Sun

One of the great all-round yoga postures for tuning and toning up; it's from Hatha yoga. Stretches long skeletal muscles. Used here as warm-up. There are twelve parts.

1 Standing, feet together, palms together in front of chest, arms bent at elbow—exhale.
2 Thumbs linked, push hands up over head, arch back—inhale.

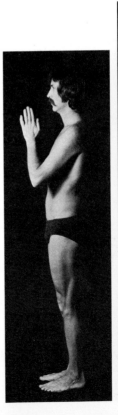
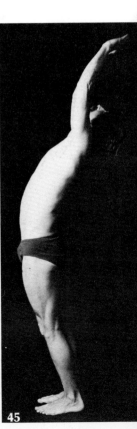

45

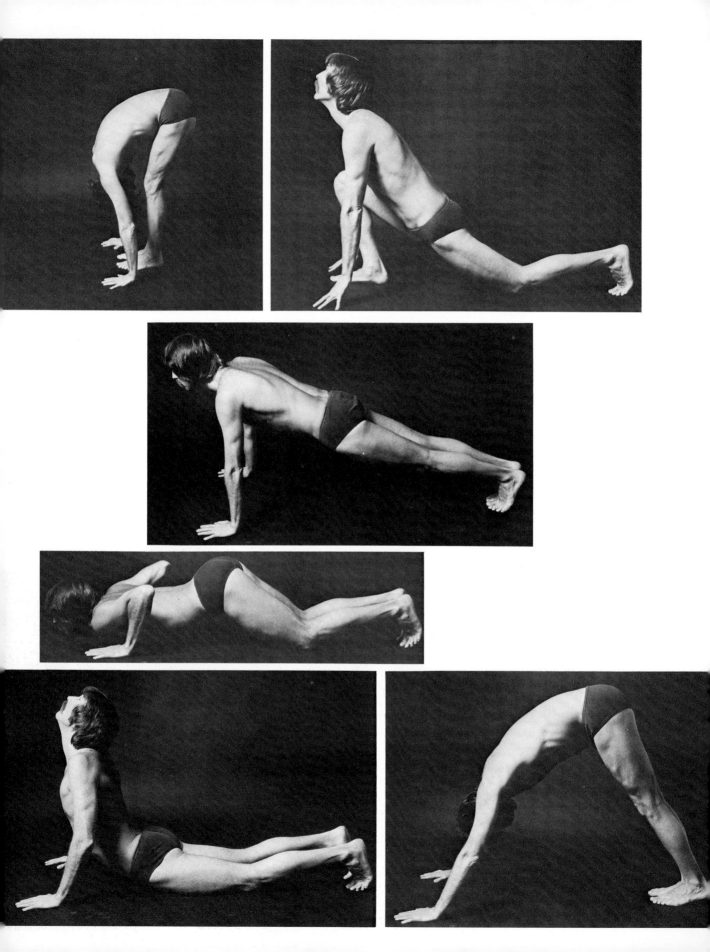

3 Bend forward at waist, drop head, hands on floor—exhale.

4 Kick left leg back, left knee on floor, arching back, head back, eyes back—inhale.

5 Right leg back, body straight, in pushup position—hold breath.

6 Drop knees, chin, chest to the floor, pelvis retracted, buttocks up—exhale.

7 Drop pelvis, push off with palms, arch back, head back, eyes back, cobra position—inhale.

8 A slight hop forward, buttocks toward sky, looking at ankles, heels pressing down toward floor—exhale.

9 Bring left foot between hands, right knee on the floor, arch back, head back, eyes back—inhale.

10 Join right foot with left, let head drop—exhale.

11 Stand, hook thumbs together, arch back—inhale.

12 Palms together in front of chest—exhale.

Start with three times going slowly; then use Salute to the Sun as an energizer or a relaxant by executing it quickly or slowly, respectively.

Remember when your body is bent forward from the vertical axis, your abdominal contractions expel air; when bent backward, your chest and belly expand and inhaling resumes.

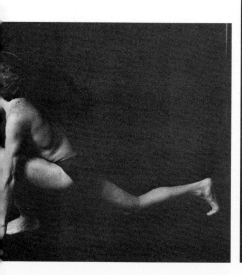
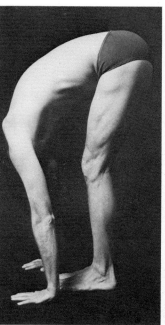
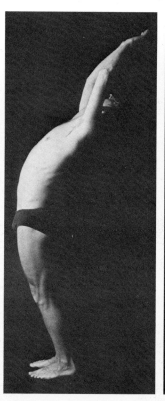
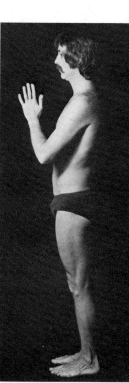

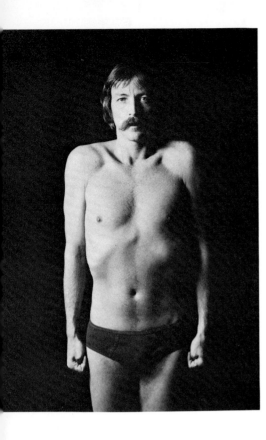

Shoulder Bounce

A Hatha yoga exercise to loosen stiff shoulders and upper back muscles.

1 Standing with feet 6 inches apart, arms at sides, wrap fingers around thumbs, making a fist.
2 Inhale, raising shoulders as high as possible.
3 Exhale, dropping shoulders, and relax.

Imagine a rod connecting shoulder to thumbs. Start with 20 breath/bounces; add two per session until you reach fifty.

Pectoral Press

Gives tone to the pectoral muscles that support breast. Helps strengthen arms. An Arica and isometrics exercise.

1 Standing with feet 6 inches apart, elbows bent, hands clasped in front of chest at shoulder level, as if to clap.
2 Right hand held by left.
3 Press heel of palms together while creating palm-to-palm pressure.
4 Inhale while pressing. Hold two counts. Exhale while releasing.

Start with ten; add ten a week until you reach fifty. Remember to keep elbows up at shoulder level.

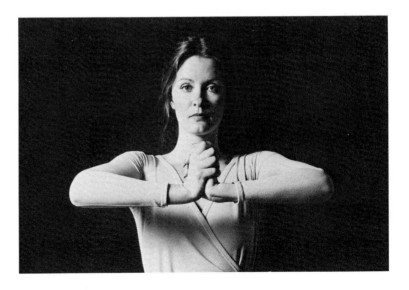

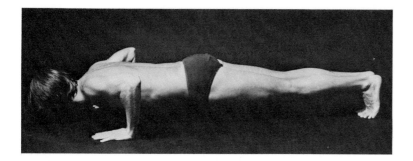

Pushup No. 1
Helps strengthen arms, chest and shoulders. Tones sagging chest. From isotonics.

1 Lying on front, palms on floor, thumbs under shoulders, toes curled onto floor.
2 Straighten arms lifting body off the floor to full extension, back straight, while inhaling.
3 Exhaling, return chest to within 1 inch from the floor, keeping body straight.

Start at four; add two each week until you reach ten.

If this regular pushup is too strenuous, strengthen arms by doing a variation.

1 Lying on front, palms on floor under shoulders.
2 Straighten arms lifting only upper body, knees stay on the floor, inhale.
3 Return to floor, exhale.

Start at four, add two each week to ten.

Trunk Lateral Bend
Light exercise, bends spine laterally while toning lateral torso and hip muscles. From Hatha yoga.

1 Standing, feet 6 inches apart, hands lightly on thighs.
2 Bend laterally from waist to right, using right hand as guide sliding down right thigh. Exhale down, inhale up to center.
3 Without stopping at the center, bend down laterally to left, using left hand as a guide. Exhale down, inhale up.

Start at ten a side, add five each week until twenty-five a side are reached. Make sure the exact line of the exercise is lateral, not forward or backward.

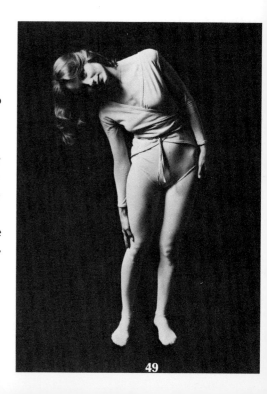

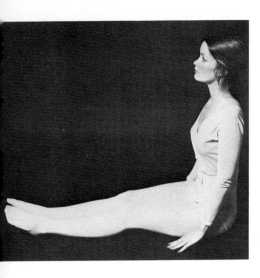

Situp No. 1

Helps strengthen and tone abdominal muscles. Prevents backaches. From isometrics.

1　On your back, arms at sides, legs together, exhale while sitting up to a vertical position, using abdominal muscles.
2　Inhale; return slowly to floor.

Start with five add three a week until you reach fifteen.

If difficult at first, elbows can be used to help you up.

Cobra

Backache caused by tension is relieved. Lower back muscles strengthened. A Hatha yoga exercise.

1　Lying on stomach, feet together, palms on floor next to shoulders.
2　Slowly inhale, and lift head, shoulders, and chest up off the floor. Body from navel to toes is on floor.
3　Take four deep breaths; during the fourth exhale and come down slowly.

Start with two; add one each week until you reach five. When moving off the floor, use lower back muscles until you cannot go any farther—then put pressure on palms against floor to get higher. When coming down, vertebra by vertebra, the head is last to turn forward, ending up with the forehead on the floor. Imagine exhalation leaving from lower back.

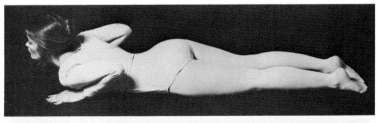

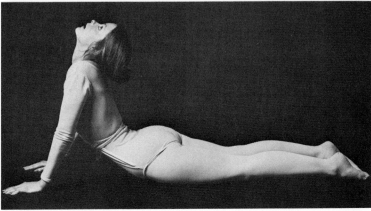

Forward Stretch

A Kundalini and Hatha yoga cleansing posture. Stimulates kidneys, pancreas and liver; excellent for diabetic patients.

1 Sit on the floor, legs extended together in front.
2 Inhale; stretch arms and torso toward sky.
3 Exhale, bending forward, holding onto the first part of your leg your hands contact from foot to knee.
4 Relax head between shoulders, close eyes, and breathe long and deep five breaths.
5 Inhale while coming up slowly and lying back on the floor in corpse pose.

Five long, deep breaths; add five each week until fifteen.

Remember to keep legs straight, back of knees on the floor. Take a few seconds to lightly bounce knees before going into Corpse Pose (see page 60).

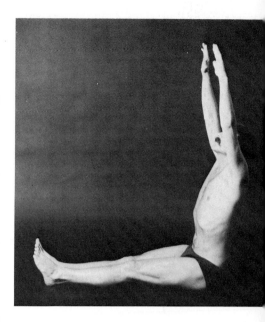

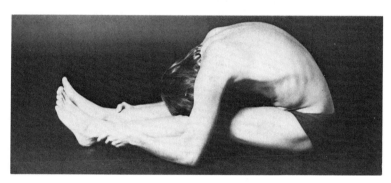

Rock Pose 60°

Stretches and massages muscles in feet, ankles, calves, and thighs. From Kundalini yoga.

1 Sit on back of legs and heels, top of feet (instep) flat on the floor.
2 Lean back 60°.

Start with five deep breaths; add three per week until you reach fourteen. Rock as you breathe.

This posture will be difficult for people who carry tension in their ankles. In seconds you may become uncomfortable. Stick with it. If it seems unbearable, put a cushion between your buttocks and legs. Imagine the pain leaving on the exhalation. It will help, at first, to rest back on arms, hands on floor.

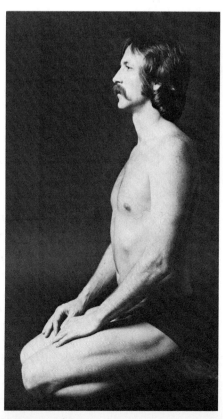

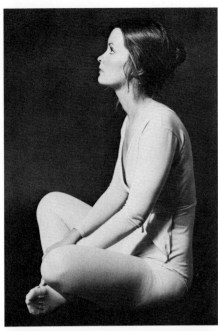

Camel Ride (Easy Pose)

Motion helps relieve pelvic and lower back tension. From Kundalini.

1 In Easy Pose, hands holding forward ankle, sitting straight.
2 Inhale, shoulders back, chest up—small of back moves forward in one movement.
3 Exhale pushing back from the small of your back—chest drops.

Get into a rhythm while doing Breath of Fire. Start with twenty breaths; add ten each each week until fifty. The movement is similar to riding a camel. Your head does not move independently in this exercise—it follows the path established by the neck and moves up and down on the same line.

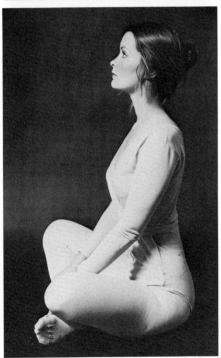

V Raise No. 1

Tones abdomen, hips, and back muscles; reduces abdominal fat. From Kundalini.

1 Sitting position, legs extended forward, lean back on elbows.
2 Lift legs to 60° from floor.
3 Look at big toes; do Breath of Fire.
4 Exhale, legs down.

Start with fifteen Breaths of Fire; add five each week until thirty.

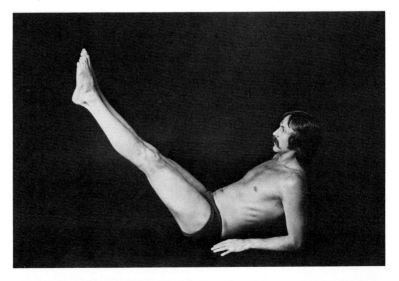

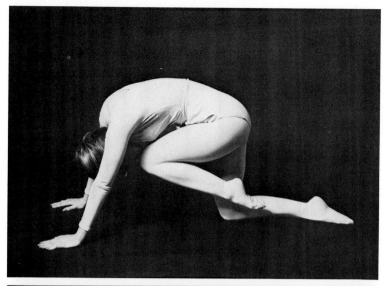

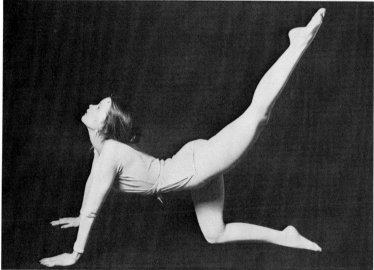

Mule Kick and Arch

Complete body stretch, especially for back and pelvis. From Kundalini.

1   On hands and knees, exhale, lifting right knee off floor and as far forward as possible while back is arching and forehead is tucked under trying to lightly meet knee.

2   Inhale, leg back, foot toward the sky; back sinks, head looking at sky. Do three.

3   Change legs.

Start with three each leg; add three each week until twelve. (Be careful not to bump knee on head.) Exercise is done in two smooth movements.

Slow Twist

Increases mobility in ankles, knees, thighs, and pelvis; helps grounding. Based on T'ai Chi.

1 Standing feet parallel, slightly wider than shoulders, with knees slightly bent, hands on hips.
2 Slowly turn to the right, moving hips and shoulders perpendicular to feet.
3 Continue turning head to the right so it is facing 180° from toes.
4 Turn head to the left facing same direction as feet.
5 Turn head same direction as shoulders and hips—and turn all together toward original position.
6 Do steps 2 through 5 on the left side.

Start with three times on each side; add one a week until six. Twisting becomes more difficult the more the knees are bent. Be aware of balance between legs. Pelvis is tucked forward slightly. Breathe and center into belly.

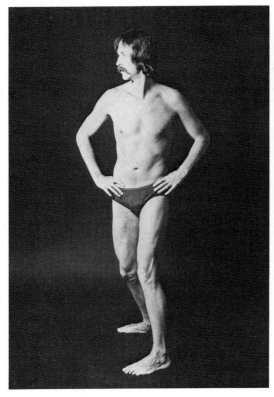 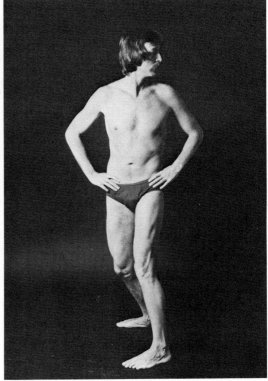

Jump Rope or Run in Place

Jump Rope (Step-over)

Increases endurance and cardiovascular and respiratory efficiency. Strengthens legs and feet. Improves grounding, coordination, and balance. From endurance training.

1 Standing with feet together, ends of rope in each hand at thigh level, middle of rope lying behind heels.
2 With a circular motion of wrists and arms, flip rope over head and back to floor. Just before rope hits floor, step over it one foot at a time, landing on the toes and ball of foot, never flat-footed.
3 Continue turning rope, stepping, jumping.

Start with fifty steps/jumps, counting each time the right foot lands as one; add twenty-five per week until you reach 150. Monitor heart rate. Rest 1 minute.

Jumping rope is an activity similar to learning to ride a bicycle. Because it takes a certain amount of balance and coordination, it can be difficult for some people at first. The rope will get caught around ankles or in toes, or you will jump on the rope instead of over it. It will take a few sessions of misses before the technique is mastered. It is helpful at first to jump without the rope, pantomiming the movement. Then add the rope.

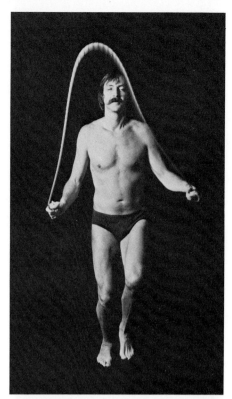

In both cases breathe through mouth into belly. Rope can be $1/4$–$1/2$ inches wide—length depends on your height. Rope used in mountain climbing is good because its weight helps keep it full as it turns.

For those who choose an alternate endurance training exercise, run in place.

Run in Place No. 1

Increases endurance and cardiovascular and respiratory efficiency. Strengthens legs, feet, arms, and shoulders. From endurance training.

1 Standing, raise each foot at least 4 inches off the floor to jog in place.

Count each time right foot hits floor as one. Start with 100; add fifty per week until you reach 250. After each 100, do ten jumping-jacks:

1 Arms at sides, feet together.
2 Swing arms upward, touching hands over head while feet jump astride.
3 Back to original position.

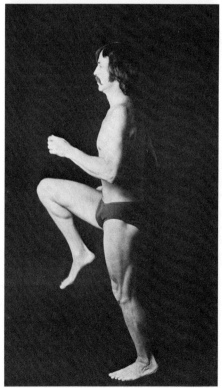

Monitor heart rate. Rest one minute before continuing. Do three Integration Breaths (see page 59).

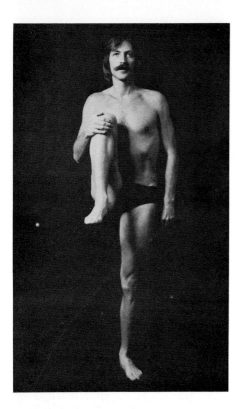

Knee to Chest
Balances, strengthens legs. Stretches inner thighs. From Kung Fu.

1 Standing, feet 6 inches apart, lift right knee to chest holding right knee with right hand, ankle with left hand. Three deep breaths into belly.
2 Repeat with left leg—three deep breaths into belly. Do three times each leg.

At first there may be difficulty getting knee near chest. Hold knee as high as you can while maintaining balance. Keep back straight.

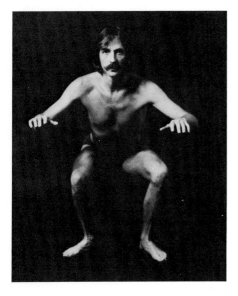

Squat Stand
Gets you in touch with your own two feet. Stimulates energy flow throughout the body. Helps open pelvic blocks. Strengthens thighs. Stretches tight muscles in legs. Adds a new sense of balance. From bioenergetics.

1 Standing, feet shoulders' width apart, slowly go into a squatting position.
2 Toes, balls of feet, and heels on floor. Adjustment in angle of feet can be made. Arms inside knees. You may have to hold on to something at first to keep your balance.
3 While aware of the entire bottom of your feet, push down, feet against the floor and slowly stand. Breathe into belly.

Start with two; add one each week, increasing to four. It may take over a week to plant your heel on the ground while squatting. Try to keep back straight. This is the most natural and healthy position for a bowel movement.

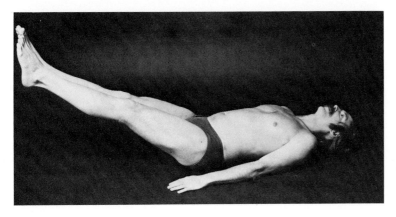

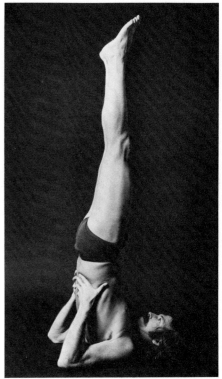

Shoulder Stand

Stimulates thyroid and parathyroid glands helping to regulate metabolism—regulates poor blood circulation and helps in reduction of abdominal fat and varicose veins. From yoga.

1 Lie on your back—feet together, arms by sides, palms down.
2 Put pressure on palms against floor to help you lift legs, feet pointing toward sky and back off floor.
3 Place your hands on back, elbows on floor, supporting back. Chin pressed against chest, concentrate on the front of neck. Take four deep breaths.
4 With hands in original position on floor, lower legs slowly.

Start with four deep breaths; add two a week until you reach ten.

This is an excellent posture for people whose jobs require them to stand or walk for long periods of time.

Fish

This is a complementary (or counter) pose to the shoulder stand—it bends the spine in the opposite direction. Stimulates thyroid glands and relieves asthma. The chest is stretched open in this position. From yoga.

1 Lying on your back, slip fingers under tops of thighs, put pressure on elbows to help arch back so you can move the top of head backward until it rests on floor. Hold for four deep breaths.
2 Come out of posture by pressing against elbows.

Start with four deep breaths; add two each week until you reach ten. When you feel secure in the Fish, place your hands on top of your thighs.

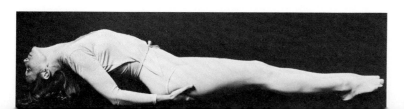

Contraction/Relaxation

Restores vitality. Done in Corpse Pose (see page 60).

1   Bring awareness to toes in your right foot; wiggle and stretch them. Spread toes apart. Relax.

2   Come up to ankle; rotate ankle, creating pressure.

3   Flex calf muscles. Relax.

4   Bring awareness to thigh. Tighten it, then more. Lift straightened leg off floor 2 inches, tighten more, then drop. Relax.

5   Roll your right leg back and forth. Become aware of left toes. Repeat technique for left leg.

6   From left thigh, take awareness to right hand. Rotate thumb and fingers; open and close palm. Stretch fingers and palm. Center of palm will rise slightly. Hold for one breath. Make a fist and rotate from wrist; create pressure for one breath. Straighten arm off floor 2 inches. Tighten fist, forearm, and upper arm as tight as you can for one breath and drop. Roll.

7   Repeat with left hand and arm.

8   Contract muscles in rectum. If done correctly, your buttocks will rise from the ground. Tighten for one breath. Exhale and relax.

9   Breathe long and deep into belly. Holding breath for three counts, push out belly. Exhale rapidly through mouth.

10 After 10 seconds of normal breathing, expand chest. Push out from inside, holding three counts; exhale rapidly.

11 Try to make shoulders meet over chest (this is only an attempt, obviously—they will never reach), holding for one breath; exhale and drop shoulders.

12 Move the muscles in your face, make ugly faces, big phony smiles to break down the tension. Imagine a paintbrush sticking out of your chin. Paint circles and figure eights on the ceiling and walls. Bring the energy into a small ball into the center of your face, trying to mash lips against nose. Inhale, exhale, while releasing contractions in face.

13 Inhale long and deep into belly. Do not contract muscles. Imagine a white vibrational wave coming in through your toes and going out the top of your head. As you imagine this wave, be aware of the different parts of your body it passes on its journey up and out the top of your head.

Contract and tense muscles as tight as you can, then release contraction and "let go" to achieve a more relaxed state. Start from your toes and think of each part of the body until you reach your head.

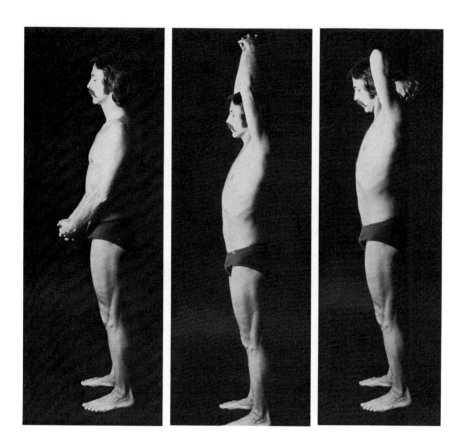

Integration Breath

Helps to integrate muscles and breathing to normal. From Arica.

1 Standing with feet 6 inches apart, clasp fingers together in front of you, letting arms relax.
2 Inhale deeply while bringing clasped hands straight over head; let the forearms fall behind the head.
3 Put a little pressure on the heels of the hands, starting the exhalation as the arms make the return trip on the same line.

As the arms move up on the inhalation, imagine them floating on the breath.

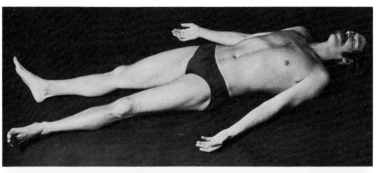

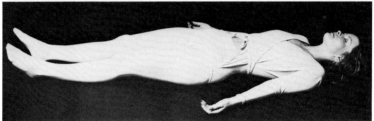

Corpse Pose

For relaxation—and to restore vitality. From yoga.

1 Lie on back, arms a few inches from body—palms up, legs spread comfortably apart.
2 Let the floor hold your body; trust it.
3 Relax all muscles.
4 Breathe into belly, causing abdomen to rise and fall.

Stay in the Corpse Pose for about 1 minute, but try not to be aware of the clock. Let your bodymind release attachment to thoughts. Listen to your body, be aware of any tension in muscles. Tighten more; release, telling the muscles to "let go" while you exhale—thus you release any attachment to that thought of muscle tension. Listen to any sounds in the room and/or outside. Again, do not become attached to the thought. No thought has any preference over any other. If the thought "I have to be at work at 9 o'clock" comes across your thought screen, drop it like any other thought. Let the thoughts pass away like clouds in the sky.

Shake

Massages and invigorates muscles; aids in relaxation.

1 Standing, shake shoulders from front to back as if out of phase with hips.
2 Shake hands and arms.
3 Shake feet and legs.

Spend a few seconds on each area you shake. Move as if you were trying to shake water off your body. For variation, open your throat and sustain an "ah" while shaking the shoulders.

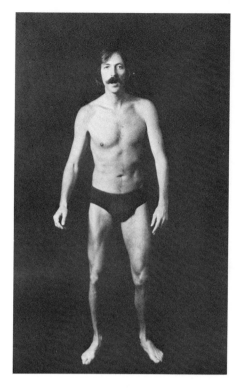

Scarab

For relaxation, increased circulation to the head and pelvis—a light stretch for thighs and ankles. Good relaxation for anal tension.

1 Palms on floor, sitting on heels, place forehead on floor in front of you, chest on thighs, palms down next to head, eyes closed.
2 Breathe long and deep into belly.

This relaxation pose will be uncomfortable until ankle and thigh tension is stretched away. Many religions use it as a position of prayer. Some say it stimulates the "third eye" (the pineal body).

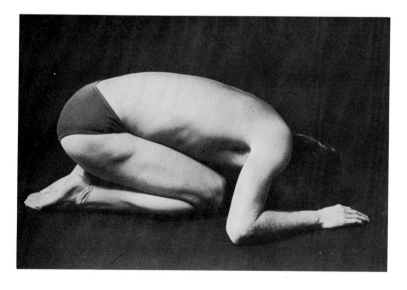

Chapter 7

Cycle II

Warm-Up:

Cooling Breath

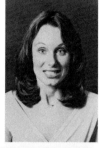

Head to
Feet Bounce

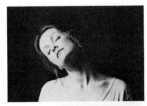

Head/Neck Roll

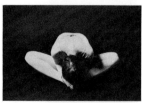

Sky/Earth
Picking Apples

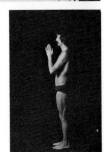

Salute to the Sun

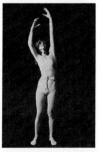

Exercises:

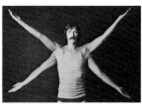

Arm Circles

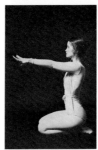

Energy Ball/
Rock Pose

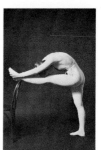

Hamstring
Stretch

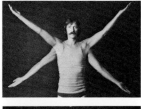

Book Lift

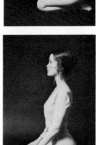

Camel Ride
(Rock Pose)

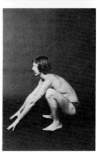

Squat Stand/
Buttocks Up

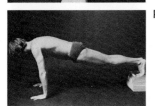

Pushup No. 2

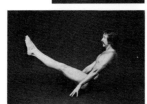

V Raise No. 2

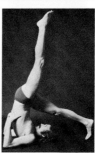

Shoulder Stand/
Leg Bounce

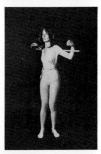

Broom
Twist

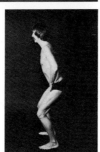

Bump/Ground
Rotation

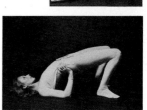

Bridge

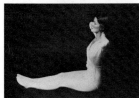

Situp No. 2

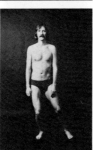

Balance
Sway

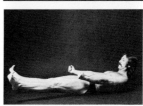

Concentration/
Relaxation (Short
Form)

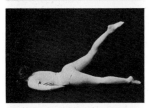

Half Locust/
Locust

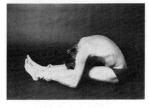

Forward Stretch/
Breath of Fire

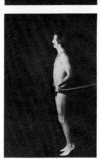

Jump Rope No. 2 or
Run in Place No. 2

Cooling Breath

Cools the system, quenches thirst, appeases hunger, and cleans blood.

1 Sitting in Easy Pose; stick your tongue a little bit out from lips.
2 Fold the tongue like a tube.
3 Inhale through the tube with a hissing sound.
4 Retain as long as comfortable.
5 Exhale slowly through both nostrils.

Do fifteen cooling breaths, two times. If you cannot fold your tongue do the variation.

Variation:

1 Fold your tongue so that the tip of it touches the upper palate.
2 Inhale air through teeth resting together, with a hissing sound.
3 Retain as long as comfortable.
4 Exhale slowly through both nostrils.

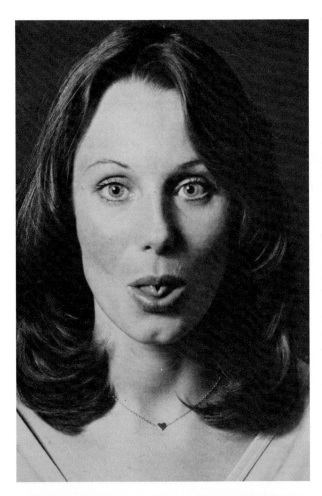
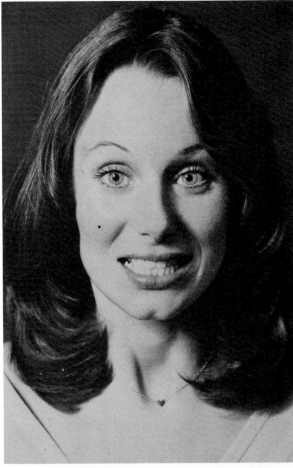

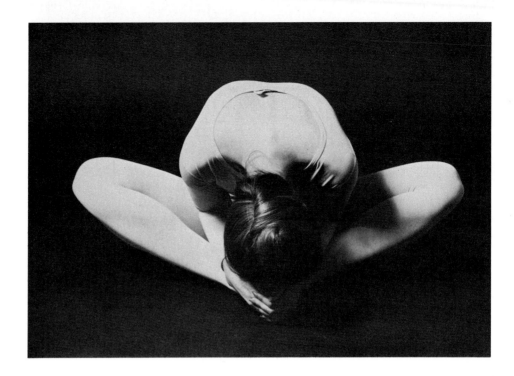

Head to Feet Bounce

This bounce loosens hip joint and groin tensions. Firms and tightens skin and muscles of inner thigh. Helps in sitting for meditation. From Kundalini.

1 Sitting on the floor, put the bottoms of your feet together.
2 Clasp your fingers together around toes.
3 Bounce knees lightly toward floor.
4 Exhale quickly through nose as knees drop toward floor; inhale as knees are brought up.
5 When finished bounces, exhale while slowly stretching head toward feet, eventually touching the two. Do three times, inhaling up and exhaling down.

Start with fifty bounces; add two per session until you reach eighty.

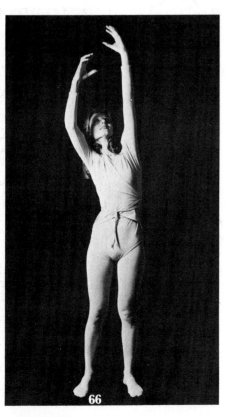

Sky/Earth Picking Apples

Warm-up stretch, loosening neck, shoulders, spine, and legs. From Arica.

1 Standing, feet at shoulder width and parallel, inhale, arms toward the sky, reaching up.
2 Exhale and slowly bring arms back down to sides. Repeat Item 1.

3 Inhale with arms up and imagine an apple tree inches above your hand. Without raising your heels off the floor reach higher and higher with each arm and shoulder, three times per side, sucking in a bit more air in each stretch.

4 Exhale, bending from waist; lightly bounce hands, arms, and shoulders toward floor three times.

5 Inhale and stretch toward sky picking apples, repeating steps 3 and 4.

After doing sequence twice, return arms to sides.

While bending, let go of neck tension—head will drop. Knees can be slightly bent.

Head/Neck Roll

Helps relieve headache and stimulates thyroid gland. (See Head/Neck Roll photograph, Cycle I, page 45.) From Kundalini.

1 Standing, feet 6 inches apart, arms by sides, drop chin to chest.

2 Rub chin lightly side to side, on chest, then roll head slowly 360° to the right three times.

3 Change direction and roll head to the left three times.

Relax shoulders, eyes closed, and concentrate on point between eyebrows. Breathe long and deep. Remember: roll slowly.

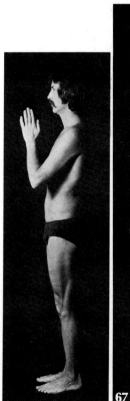
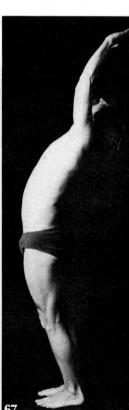

Salute to the Sun

One of the great all-round yoga postures for tuning and toning up; it's from Hatha yoga. Stretches long skeletal muscles. Used here as warm-up. There are twelve parts.

1 Standing, feet together, palms together in front of chest, arms bent at elbow—exhale.

2 Thumbs linked, push hands up over head, arch back—inhale.

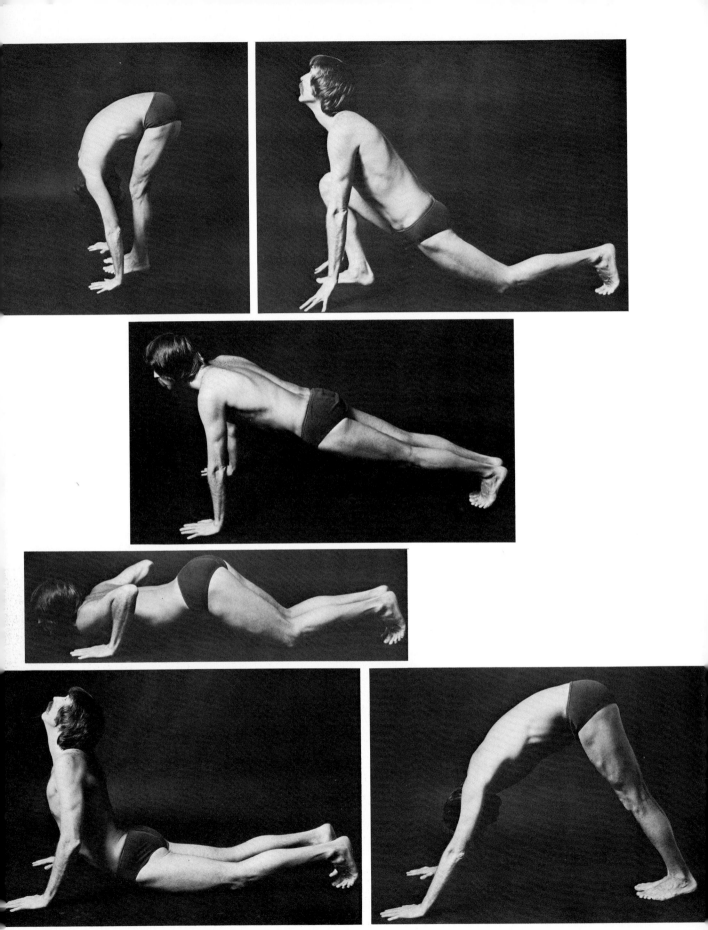

3   Bend forward at waist, drop head, hands on floor—exhale.
4   Kick left leg back, left knee on floor, arching back, head back, eyes back—inhale.
5   Right leg back, body straight, in pushup position—hold breath.
6   Drop knees, chin, chest to the floor, pelvis retracted, buttocks up—exhale.
7   Drop pelvis, push off with palms, arch back, head back, eyes back, cobra position—inhale.
8   A slight hop forward, buttocks toward sky, looking at ankles, heels pressing down toward floor—exhale.
9   Bring left foot between hands, right knee on the floor, arch back, head back, eyes back—inhale.
10 Join right foot with left, let head drop—exhale.
11 Stand, hook thumbs together, arch back—inhale.
12 Palms together in front of chest—exhale.

Start with three times doing slowly, then use Salute to the Sun as an energizer or a relaxant by executing it quickly or slowly, respectively.

Remember when your body is bent forward from the vertical axis, your abdominal contractions expel air; when bent backward, your chest and belly expand and inhaling resumes.

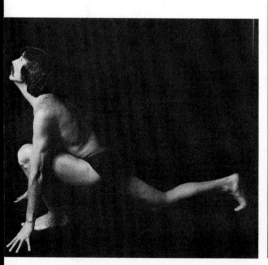
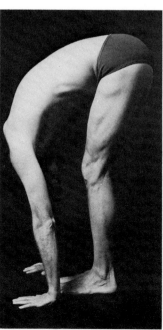
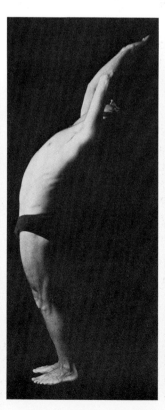
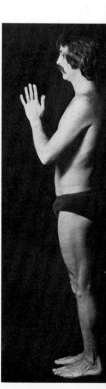

Arm Circles

Helps relieve tension in shoulders and neck; strengthens shoulders and arms. From isotonics.

1 Standing with feet at shoulder width, arms horizontal, parallel with floor, palms facing sky.
2 Describe small circles, moving arms back to front.
3 Increase the size of the circle as much as possible in ten circles.
4 Decrease size of circle until arms become parallel with floor in tenth circle (starting point).
5 Reverse the direction of arm swings.

Do not drop arms between steps 4 and 5. Breathe into belly.

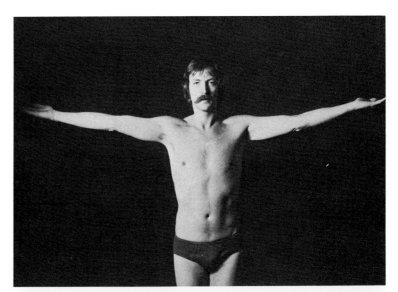

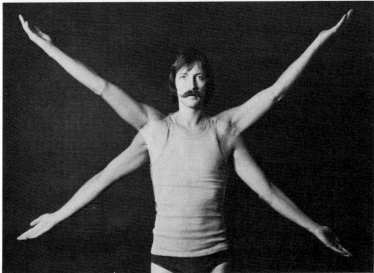

Book Lift

Improves tone in pectoral muscles. From isotonics.

1   Lie on back, arms extended on ground, holding one book
    in each hand.
2   Inhale slowly, raising books to the center of the chest,
    without bending elbows; press together.
3   Exhale slowly, lower books, elbows locked in original
    position.

Start with ten; add ten each week until you reach forty.
Eventually you will use this book and three others approximately the same size, two in each hand. You can add weight,
but never make it too heavy. You are exercising toward muscle
tone, not weight-lifting strength.

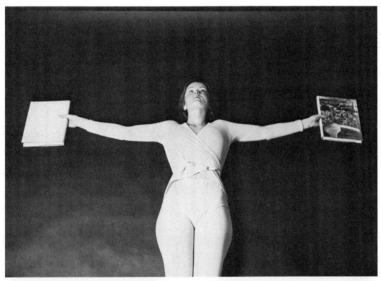

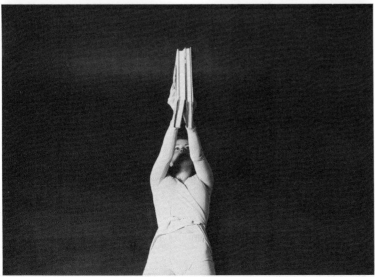

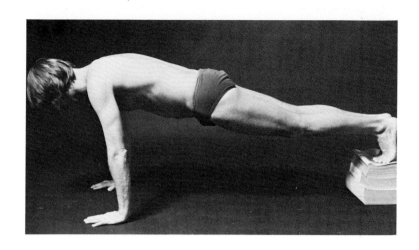

Pushup No. 2

Helps strengthen arms, chest, and shoulder muscles; tones sagging chest. From isotonics.

In pushup position, place feet on a raised platform 12 to 18 inches high. Start with ten; add two each week until you reach sixteen. A couch, low table, or a box can be used for the platform.

Broom Twist

Moves slumping shoulders back toward their natural position while making the spine more elastic. It also stimulates the spinal nerves and ligaments attached to the vertebrae.

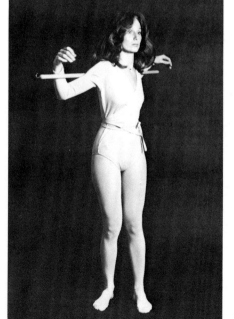

1   Standing, feet apart and parallel, put broom handle behind neck a few inches below shoulders, hands draped over ends of handle, wrists resting on handle.
2   Stiff straight legs means you are locked and immobile—so bend slightly at the knees.
3   Inhale while swinging around to the right, exhale back through center.
4   Inhale while swinging around to the left, exhale back through center.

The breathing and swinging movement is done in a smooth rhythmical motion. There is no stopping between right and left side swings. It takes a little practice to integrate breath and movement. Swing head and eyes around with torso—eyes looking to the far corner on each side.

Start with ten swings to each side; add ten each week until you reach forty.

Variation:

1   Same as Item 1 above.
2   Bend forward at waist.
3   Twist to right pointing the right arm toward left foot.
4   Twist to left pointing left arm to right foot.

Breathing is the same as above.

Situp No. 2
Helps strengthen abdominal muscles and prevents backaches.

1   Lying on your back, legs together, fingers interlaced behind neck, exhale sitting up to a vertical position using abdominal muscles.
2   Inhale as you return to floor.

Start with ten; add five each week until you reach twenty-five.

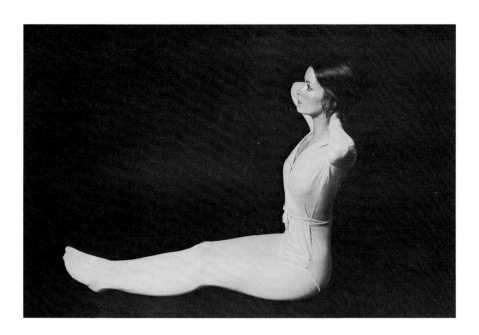

Half Locust/Locust

Stimulates circulation in spine and abdominal organs. Strengthens muscles in lower back; firms thighs, hips, and buttocks. From yoga.

1   Lying face down, chin on the floor, fists under pelvis.
2   Inhale, raising right leg from hip as high off floor as possible; retain breath for three counts.
3   Exhale, moving right leg slowly down to floor.
4   Repeat with left leg.
5   Inhale with both legs off the floor. Retain breath for three counts.
6   Exhale with both legs moving slowly down to floor.

Start raising each leg once and both legs once; add one each week until you can raise each leg four times. Fists are relaxed, not tight (the shape is important), thumbs side by side with index fingers.

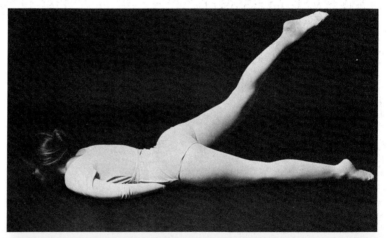

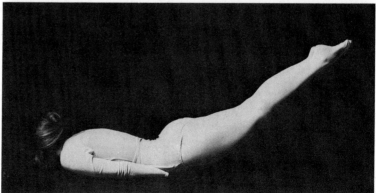

Forward Stretch/Breath of Fire

A Kundalini and Hatha yoga cleansing posture which stimulates kidneys, pancreas, liver, and stomach.

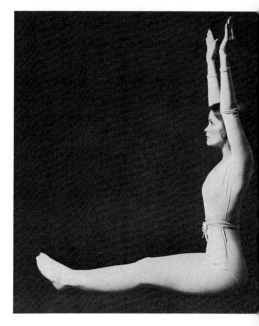

1 Sitting on the floor with back straight, legs extended together in front.
2 Inhale; stretch arms and torso toward sky.
3 Exhale bending forward, gripping the lower part of your leg, your hands contacting your leg from foot to knee.
4 Relax head between shoulders, close eyes, and breathe long and deep five breaths.
5 Breath of Fire fifteen times, inhale; retain breath five seconds.
6 Exhale, while using the muscles in your hands and arms to pull head ever so slightly forward and down toward your knees by pulling on your legs.
7 Inhale, then continue Breath of Fire fifteen times. Inhale; retain breath five seconds.
8 Repeat step 6.
9 Inhale, while coming up slowly and lying back on the floor in Corpse Pose.

Start with fifteen Breaths of Fire; add five each week until you reach thirty.

Remember to keep legs straight, backs of knees on the floor. Take a few seconds to lightly bounce knees and circle feet from ankles to alleviate stiffness before going into Corpse Pose.

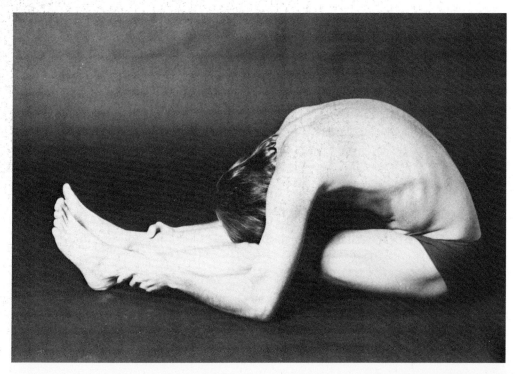

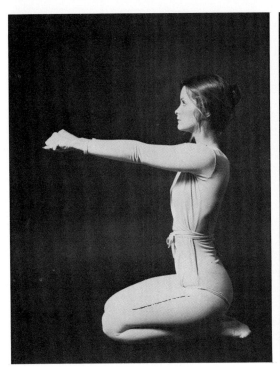 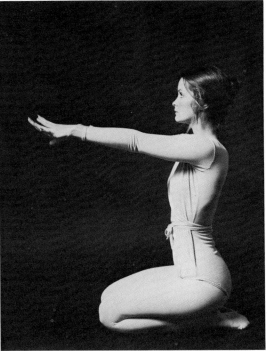

Energy Ball/Rock Pose

Stimulates and strengthens wrist, forearms, hands and shoulders. From Kundalini.

1   Sitting in rock pose extend arms and hands to the front horizontal, palms down.
2   Open and close palms as if flicking off something from fingers. Do ten times.
3   Turn right palm up; repeat ten times.
4   Reverse—left palm up, right palm down. Open and close ten times.
5   Both palms up, open and close ten times.

6   Keep arms up, fingers extended, palms facing each other. Bring palms to 6 inches apart.
7   Concentrate on the space between hands—the Energy Ball—while moving the Ball in toward chest at heart level. Drop hands.

Start with ten times in each position; add five each week until you can do twenty.

Hands have healing power. Watch what your hands do when you have a stomach ache, headache, or pain in side or anywhere on or in your body. Hands hold it. Hands are drawn to aches and pain. Work on directing energy through your hands; the ability to heal can develop.

Camel Ride/(Rock Pose)

Motion works on relieving pelvic and lower back tension. Stretches thighs and ankles. Helps open pelvic blocks, aids in energy flow. From Kundalini.

1 Rock pose, knees on floor, sitting on heels, back straight.
2 Inhale—shoulders back, chest up, small of back moves forward in one movement.
3 Exhale push back from the small of your back—chest drops.

Get into a rhythm of fire breathing. Start with thirty breaths; add ten each week up to sixty. If there is too much tension at ankles, put a cushion between floor and ankles or buttocks and ankles. Remember that your head does not move independently.

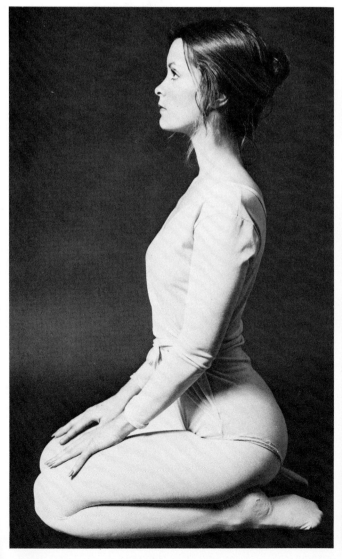
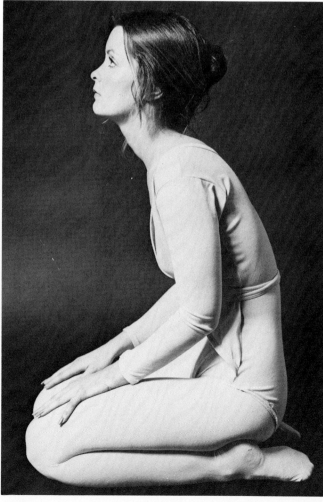

V Raise No. 2

Tones abdominal, thigh, and back muscles. From Kundalini.

1 In sitting position, legs extended, place fingertips (arms extended downward) on floor adjacent to outside of thighs. Lean back 45°.

2 Lift legs to 45° from floor.

3 Look at big toes; do fire breathing.

Start with twenty; add five each week until you reach thirty-five.

Slight adjustment will be made by hands when leaning back.

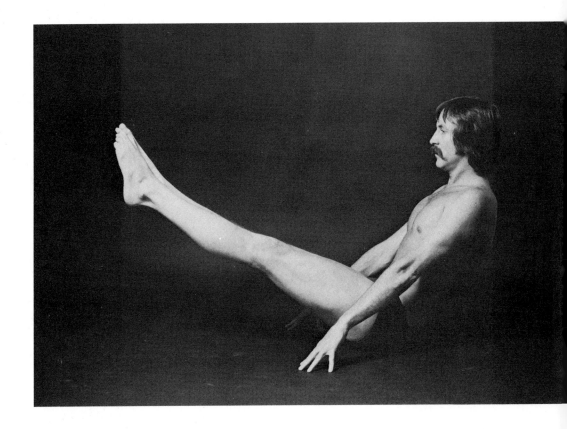

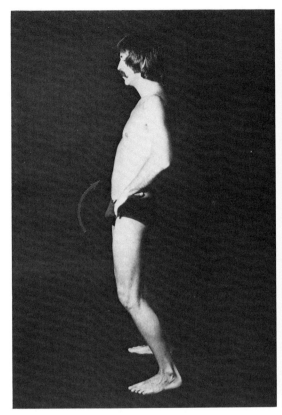 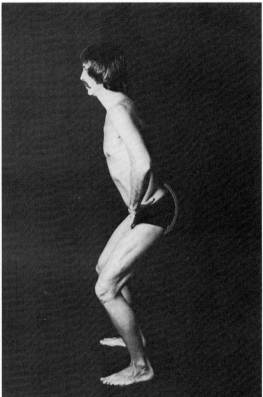

Bump/Ground Rotation

Adds flexibility to pelvis, stretches lower back, aids in grounding, strengthens thighs. From bioenergetics.

1 Standing, feet at shoulder width and parallel, knees slightly bent, hands on hips.
2 Exhale; do a semisquat, bend knees, pushing buttocks back.
3 Inhale; tuck buttocks under, moving pelvis forward and up into standing position.

Start with ten; add five each week until you reach twenty-five. Breathe into belly while moving; continue rotation of pelvis.

This exercise is hard to do for many people, more for psychological than physical reasons. Our inhibitions seem to interfere with this exercise. Enjoy your body and the flexibility and range of movement it is capable of.

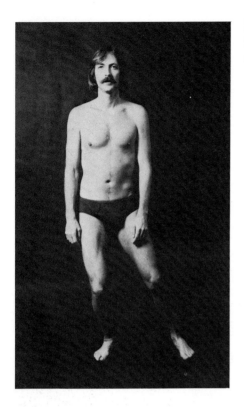

Balance Sway

Strengthens calves, thighs, and hips, while restoring fluidity to ankles and tendons. A T'ai Chi technique.

1   Standing, feet at shoulder width and parallel, bend knees slightly forward.
2   Slowly shift weight laterally onto right foot and leg, right knee directly in line over foot. Concentrate and breathe five deep breaths into the point three fingers' width below your navel.
3   Slowly push off the right foot onto the left. As you make the move across stay on the same horizontal line. Breathe as in step 2.
4   Use (and be aware of) the muscles on the inside of your right leg to go back to right leg and right foot. Experience the shifting of weight as light and heavy. Now the right side is heavy.
5   Dip lower, a little deeper into right leg. Take five deep breaths, lift (light) left leg off floor to experience balance for a moment.
6   Repeat on left leg.
7   Shift balance to the right leg; experience inside right leg pulling, left leg pushing. Dip deeper into leg for a count of five deep breaths.
8   Repeat on left leg.
9   Massage legs by shaking.

Start at three breaths per leg; add three each week until you attain twelve. Keep centering on the point below your navel throughout the exercise and be aware of the position of the parts of your body. A mirror helps. There is a feeling of being connected to the ground. Get the feeling of being heavy in the leg that is connected to the ground and light in the other leg. The degrees of this light-heavy relationship are constantly changing. When dipping into one leg in this exercise, you are 95%–100% heavy in the leg connected to the ground, depending on whether you lift the light foot off the ground. The transfer from one leg to another makes it seem as if you were pouring water from one leg to the other.

Jump Rope No. 2 or Run in Place No. 2

Jump Rope No. 2

Increases endurance and cardiovascular and respiratory efficiency. Strengthens legs and feet. Improves grounding, coordination, and balance. From endurance training.

1 Jump Rope position.
2 Jump off both feet together, landing initially on toes, then balls of feet, finally on heels, in sequence—all with knees slightly bent, feet lightly resting onto heels.

Start with 150 jumps; add twenty-five per week until 250. Monitor heart rate. Rest 1 minute. When landing on toes and balls of feet, the weight of this action coming into your heels should not cause any concussion to legs and knees. It is gentle. If it is difficult using rope, pantomime first. Jump off floor, just high enough to clear rope.

The graceful, agile, and supremely self-confident Masai and Samburu warriors of East Africa leap from a standing position straight up into the air, arms held tightly into their sides. They land on the toes-balls-heels (in sequence) of both feet. This dance/sport is a competitive game that is played spontaneously throughout the day.

Instead of this exercise you may do Run in Place No. 2.

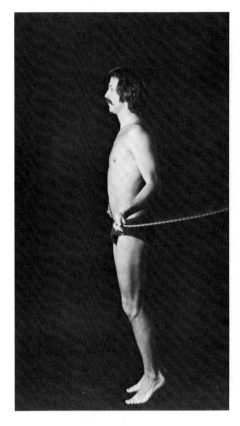

Run in Place No. 2

Increases endurance, cardiovascular and respiratory efficiency. Strengthens legs, feet, arms, and shoulders.

Standing, raise each foot at least 5 inches off the floor to jog in place. Start with 250; add fifty per week until you reach 400. After each 100, do ten jumping-jacks. Rest 1 minute before you continue program. Move your body—either walk or shake. Monitor heart rate.

Instead of this exercise, you may do Jump Rope No. 2.

Hamstring Stretch

Stretches and stimulates thigh and leg muscles, particularly hamstring muscles in back of thigh. A Kung Fu exercise.

1 Standing, place heel of right leg on a secure table, chair, or fence so the right leg is extended 90°.

2 Hold hands onto ankle of extended leg; relax head to knee.

3 Reverse legs.

Start with twenty Breaths of Fire on each leg. Add ten breaths a week until you reach sixty.

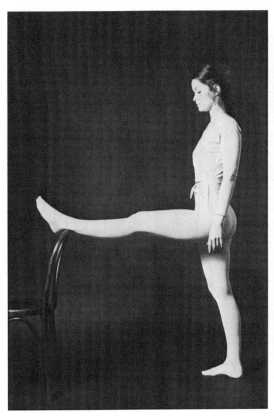
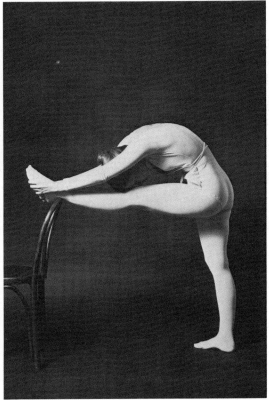

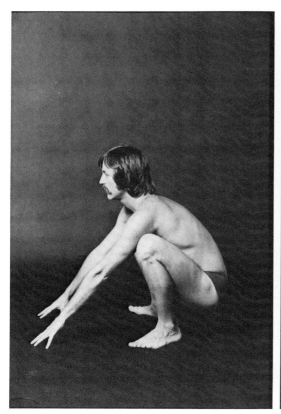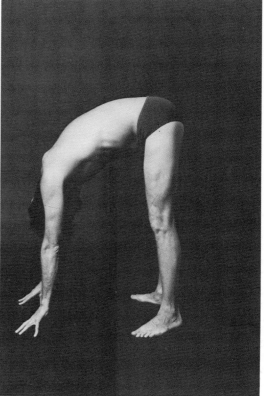

Squat Stand/Buttocks Up

Strengthens legs, stretches muscles in back of legs, develops grounding, helps release pelvic blocks. A bioenergetics exercise.

1 Sit in the squat position, entire foot on floor, arms between knees and extended, placing fingertips on floor.
2 Inhale as buttocks "stand up" toward the sky; hold two counts.
3 Exhale, sitting back down into squat position. Do twice.
4 Do squat stand (see page 56) four times after the stretches.

Start with two stretch-ups; add one each week until you reach four. Remember to drop head when inhaling. Fingertips remain on floor. Legs will eventually straighten.

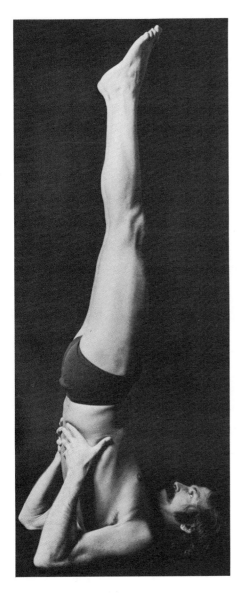

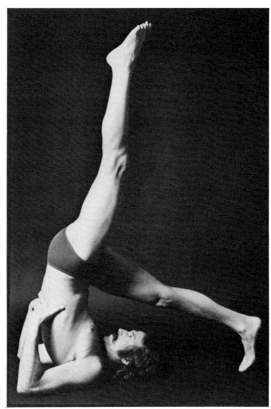

Shoulder Stand/Leg Bounce

Has positive effects of shoulder stand—plus an added stretch on muscles and added nerve toning to back of leg.

1 Go into a shoulder stand for ten breaths.
2 Slowly lower right leg (keep straight) down behind you and gently bounce your foot toward the floor three times.
3 Raise leg up and do left leg.

Alternate legs two times; add one alternation each week until you reach five. Remember to bounce gently, keeping leg straight. This will prepare you for the Plough (page 141).

Bridge

This is another pose which is complementary to the shoulder stand—it bends the spine in the opposite direction. Improves balance. From yoga.

1 From the shoulder stand, bend knees and slowly bring one leg forward followed closely by the other.
2 Place feet on the floor while hands are still holding back. Change hand position to thumbs facing each other at small of back.

Start with four full breaths into the chest; add two each week until you reach ten. You may lose your balance and fall a few inches to the floor or your arms may collapse—don't be discouraged. After a few sessions you will be in balance. If you are lying on the floor, push your pelvis up, bracing your arms by placing your elbows on the floor.

Special consideration for wrists: when first learning the transition movement from shoulder stand to Bridge, change hand position to thumbs facing each other before making movement in step 2.

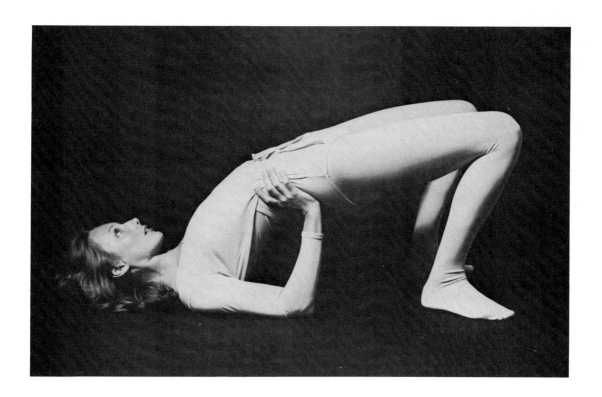

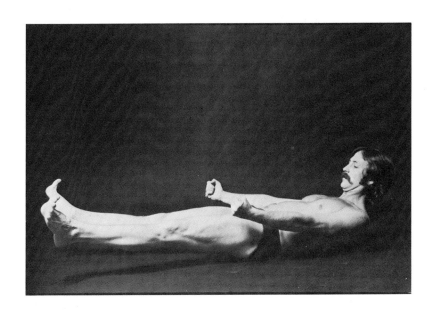

Contraction/Relaxation—Short Form

Restores vitality. (See directions on page 58.) From yoga.

1 Lying on ground, inhale; contract and straighten arm and leg muscles while lifting them off the floor 2 inches. Make tight fists and tighten face muscles. Hold for five counts.

2 Exhale, release contraction. Drop arms and legs, "let go," and breathe long and deep. You will feel relaxed and invigorated almost immediately.

Chapter 8

Cycle III

Warm-Up:

Complete Breath

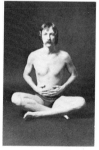

Egyptian Stretch

Sky/Earth Picking Apples/Touch Heels

Neck Stretch

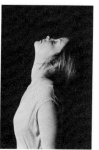

Salute to the Sun

Exercises:

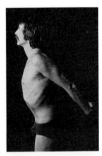

Shoulder
Roll

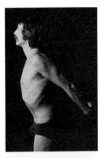

Pushup
Sleeve

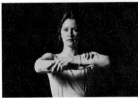

Pushup
No. 3

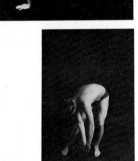

Ax Twist

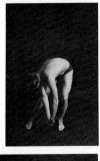

Situp Knees
to Chest

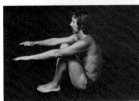

Bow

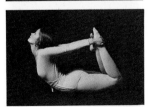

Forward
Stretch
Groin

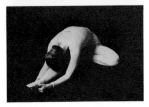

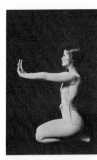

Wrists Up/Down
(Rock Pose)

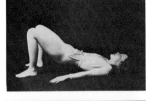

Pelvic Bounce

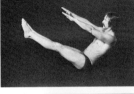

V Raise No. 3

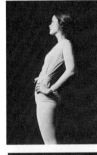

Hip Swing

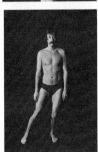

Lateral Walk

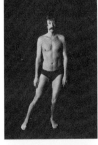

Jump Rope

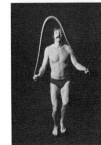

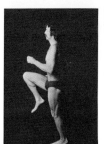

Run in Place
No. 3

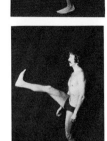

Pendulum Kick

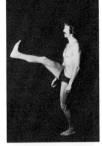

Masai Stand

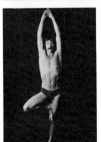

Head Stand

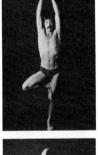

Lion

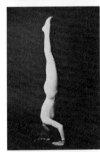

Contraction/
Relaxation

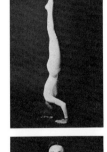

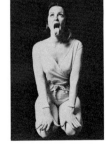

Complete Breath

Restores vitality.

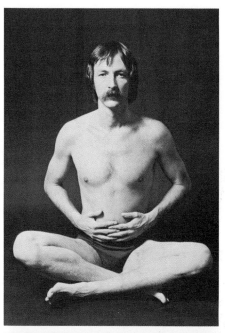

1 Sit in Easy Pose, keeping the head, neck, and trunk in a straight line.
2 Place hands over navel at first to get the feeling of the diaphragm expanding and contracting.
3 Inhale through nose, first filling the lower part of the lungs as the diaphragm descends—exert a gentle pressure on the walls of the abdomen, as if you were breathing into your hands.
4 Fill the middle part of the lungs, pushing out the lower ribs and chest. Feel and see this area expand.
5 Fill the higher portion of the lungs, expanding the chest. The abdomen will be slightly drawn in. At the end of the inhalation, while air is still being drawn in, slightly raise the shoulders, allowing air to pass into the smaller upper lobes of the lungs. Do not force the shoulders back—lift them up.
6 Retain a few counts. (Do not retain the first week.) Do this part of the exercise 3 seconds to 1 minute.
7 Exhale slowly, drawing the abdomen upward and back toward the spinal column.
8 At the end of exhalation, immediately inhale again. Breathe normally after one round of three complete breaths.

Start with three rounds.

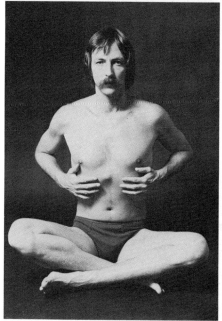

The Complete Breath may seem awkward in the beginning, especially if you haven't mastered deep breathing, but it is a natural way of breathing which practice will soon make habitual. It will be helpful to stand or sit up right in front of a mirror during this exercise, placing your hands over each part of the body to feel the expansion of abdomen, ribs, and chest as the breath flows in. Concentrate on a smooth, even flow as you inhale and exhale through the nose.

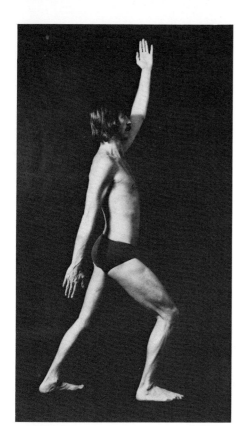

Egyptian Stretch

Stretches and strengthens shoulder, back, thigh, and leg muscles. Develops coordination and grounding.

1 Stand with feet 6 inches apart.
2 Inhale as you lunge the right leg forward, simultaneously raising left arm straight over head and stretching right arm down and back.
3 Exhale; return to standing position.
4 Repeat with left leg forward.

Count one for each time right leg is forward. Start with three; add three per week until you reach nine.

The lunge is a long stride forward. Feel the effect of the stretch in legs and shoulders.

Sky/Earth Picking Apples/Touch Heels

Warm-up stretch. Same benefits as Sky/Earth Picking Apples (see page 66) with extra waist and spine stretch. *Note*: While bending, legs are kept straight.

1 While standing, feet at shoulder width and parallel, inhale, arms toward the sky, reaching up.
2 Exhale and slowly bring arms back down to sides. Repeat once.
3 Inhale with arms up and imagine an apple tree inches above your hand. Without raising your heels off the floor reach higher and higher alternately with each arm and shoulder, three times a side, sucking in a bit more air with each stretch.
4 Exhale, bending from waist; lightly bounce hands, arms, shoulders, and head toward floor three times. When bending from waist touch hands to floor behind heels.
5 Inhale and stretch toward sky picking apples, repeating steps 3 and 4 twice.

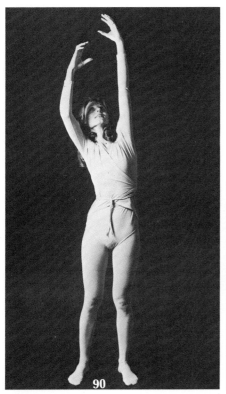

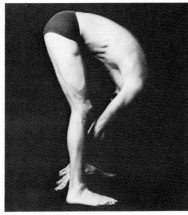

Neck Stretch

Stretches neck muscles; relieves tension and headaches. From yoga.

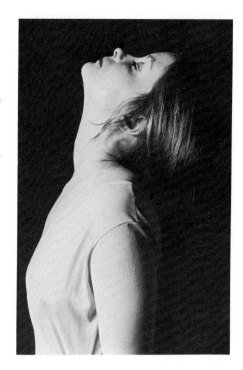

1 Standing with feet 6 inches apart, arms at sides, lower chin toward chest. Rest in this position for three long deep breaths.
2 Slowly roll head to left shoulder position. Rest for three long deep breaths.
3 Slowly roll head to back position. Rest for three long deep breaths.
4 Slowly roll head to right shoulder position. Rest for three long deep breaths.
5 Slowly roll head to forward chest position. Rest for three long deep breaths.
6 Reverse direction (right–back–left–chest) for three long deep breaths each.

Breathe into belly.

Salute to the Sun

See page 39. One of the great all-round yoga postures for tuning and toning up; it's from Hatha yoga. Stretches long skeletal muscles. Used here as warm-up. There are twelve parts.

1 Standing, feet together, palms together in front of chest, arms bent at elbow—exhale.
2 Thumbs locked, push hands up over head, arch back—inhale.
3 Bend forward at waist, drop head, hands on floor—exhale.
4 Kick left leg back, left knee on floor, arching back, head back, eyes back—inhale.
5 Right leg back, body straight, in pushup position—hold breath (see photograph).
6 Drop knees, chin, chest to the floor, pelvis retracted, buttocks up—exhale.
7 Drop pelvis, push off with palms, arch back, head back, eyes back, cobra position—inhale (see photograph).
8 A slight hop forward, buttocks toward sky, looking at ankles, heels pressing down toward floor—exhale.
9 Bring left foot between hands, right knee on the floor, arch back, head back, eyes back—inhale.
10 Join right foot with left, let head drop—exhale.

11   Stand, hook thumbs together, arch back—inhale.

12   Palms together in front of chest—exhale.

Start with three times going slowly, then use Salute to the Sun as an energizer or a relaxant by executing it either quickly or slowly, respectively.

Remember when your body is bent forward from the vertical axis, your abdominal contractions expel air; when bent backward, your chest and belly expand and inhaling resumes.

Shoulder Roll

Stretches shoulders and upper back muscles; helps coordination. An Arica technique.

1   Standing with feet at shoulder width and parallel, clasp hands together behind buttocks.

2   Inhale, moving clasped hands up spinal column, shoulders rotating forward.

3   Exhale, pushing hands away from body, straightening arms, arching back, shoulders stretching back.

4   Hands return to original position at buttocks.

Start with four; add two each week until you reach ten.

Get into the rhythm of continuous circular motion of the rotation.

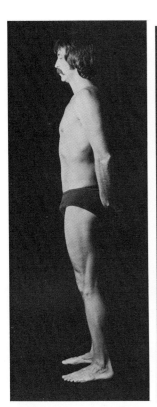 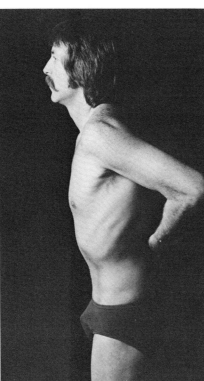 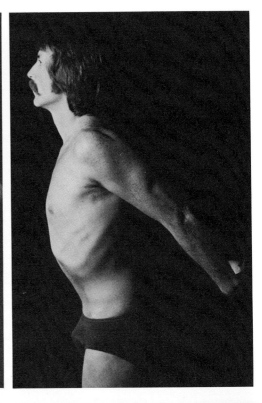

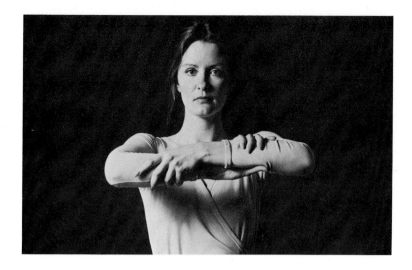

Pushup Sleeve

Helps tone pectoral muscles. From isometrics.

1 Stand with feet 6 inches apart and parallel; each hand grasps the other forearm near elbow.
2 Without letting go of the light grip, make a movement as if you are pushing up your sleeve (or skin) toward your elbow; hold for one count.

Start with twenty; add ten each week up to fifty. Keep arms shoulder height for maximum benefits. Add a bit more pressure at the end of the pushup motion. Inhale on press.

Pushup No. 3

Strengthens arm, chest, and shoulder muscles; tones sagging chest. From isometrics.

In pushup position, feet on a raised platform 24–30 inches high, do pushup exercise.

Start with sixteen; add two each week until you reach twenty-two. Make sure platform is secure before putting your weight on it. Use couch, chair, box, or part of bed.

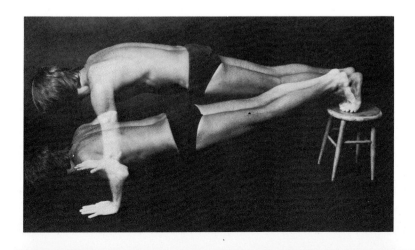

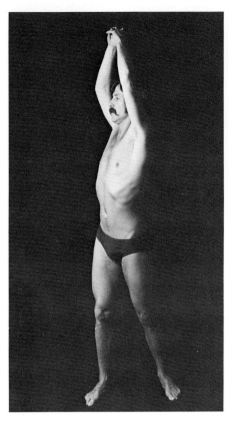

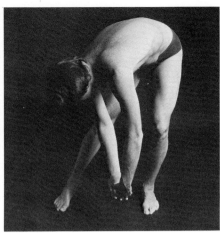

Ax Twist

Stretches spine, tones lateral trunk and hip muscles, strengthens leg muscles, helps grounding. From Arica.

1 Standing, feet at shoulder width and parallel, knees slightly bent.
2 Inhale, with hands clasped over head as if holding an ax.
3 Turn your body to the right without moving feet and swing the ax down as you exhale and follow through.
4 Inhale, swinging up to the right along the same line you swung down.
5 Turn to the left without moving feet and swing the ax down as you exhale.

Start with four on each side; add two per week until you reach ten. Bend knees further as you swing down. Feel feet in touch with floor. Follow through, hands lower than knees.

Situp Knees to Chest

Tones abdominal muscles, develops coordination. An isotonic technique.

1 Lying on back, arms extended on floor behind head, feet together.
2 Exhale, sitting up, bringing knees to chest, arms extended straight forward, parallel to floor.
3 Inhale, back to flat-on-the-floor position.

Start with twenty; add five each week up to forty.

Variation: Keep feet off the floor when sitting up. It's harder to do at first, but further strengthens abdominal muscles and coordination.

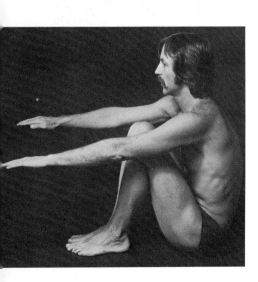

Bow

Aids digestion, helps relieve constipation and gastrointestinal disorders. Strengthens back muscles. From yoga.

1   Lying on your stomach, knees bent, legs a few inches apart, raise and grab hold of right ankle with right hand, left with left.
2   Inhale, pulling against the ankles, raise head, chest, and thighs off the floor, body resting on pelvis.
3   Retain the breath for five counts and slowly come down, letting go of ankles.

Start with one; add one a week until you reach four.

At first it may be difficult to get thighs off the ground. Don't be discouraged—with the right amount of effort, anything you want will happen. This pose has the combination of effects of the Cobra and Locust Poses.

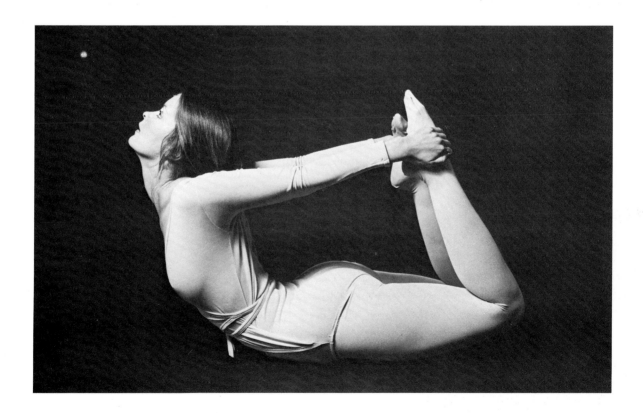

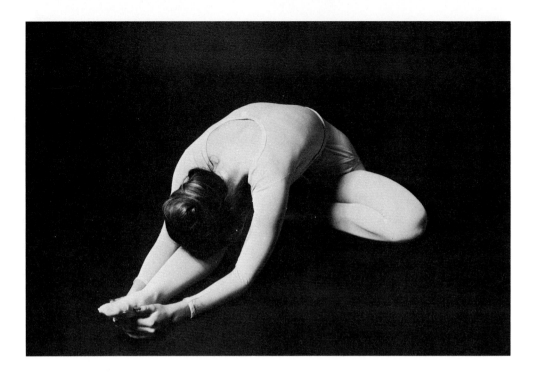

Forward Stretch Groin

Benefits of forward stretch, plus additional stretching of inner thigh and buttocks. From Kundalini.

1 Sitting on floor, legs extended.
2 Bend right knee placing right foot against left inner thigh.
3 Inhale, stretch arms and torso toward sky.
4 Exhale, bending forward and holding onto the first part of your leg your hands contact.
5 Relax head between shoulders; close eyes and breathe long and deep ten breaths.
6 Inhale while coming up slowly.
7 Change legs and repeat.

Start with ten long deep breaths; add five each week to reach twenty-five. Take a few seconds to lightly bounce knees before going into Corpse Pose. This ultimate forward stretch is head touching knees, elbows on floor.

Wrists Up/Down (Rock Pose)

Stimulates and strengthens wrists, forearms, and shoulders, while stretching thighs and ankles. From Kundalini.

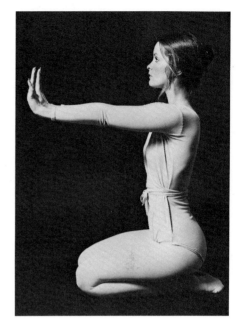

1 Sitting in rock pose, extend arms and hands to horizontal position, hands open, palms down.
2 Lift hands up, bending at wrists, fingers toward sky.
3 Drop hands, fingers pointing to floor.

Start with twenty-five; add five each week to reach forty. Count each "up" as one. Breathe into belly. Feel pressure at wrists.

Pelvic Bounce

Helps energy flow into pelvic area. From bioenergetics.

1 Lying on your back, knees up, feet close to buttocks, arms by your side.
2 Raise buttocks off the floor 3 to 4 inches.
3 Bounce pelvis gently toward sky without touching the floor.

Start with fifteen bounces; add five each week until you reach thirty. Breathe through mouth into belly.

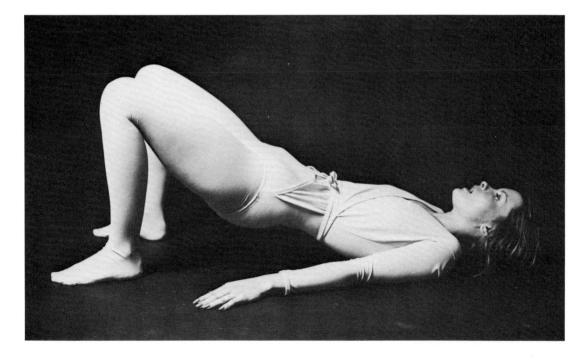

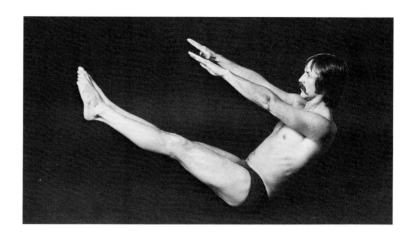

V Raise No. 3
Tones abdominal, thigh and lower back muscles, develops balance. From Kundalini.

1 In sitting position, legs extended forward, place fingertips next to the outside of thighs. Lean back 45°.
2 Lift legs to 45° from floor, then remove fingers from floor, arms parallel with leg. Balance.
3 Look at big toes; do fire breathing.

Start with fifteen; add five each week until you reach thirty.

Hip Swing
Integrates breathing, movement, and feeling; helps abdominal tone. From bioenergetics.

1 Standing, feet 6 inches apart, hands on hips, with thumbs facing to rear.
2 Tilt pelvis forward, then slowly swing hips in a horizontal circle to the right. Breathe into belly as you move.
3 Change direction to left.

While standing straight, imagine your body, head to feet, as opposite poles of an axis, and slowly swing your hips around this axis. Your hands can help by tilting hips forward in the front position and retracting pelvis in back position. Start with five swings in each direction; add five each week until you reach twenty.

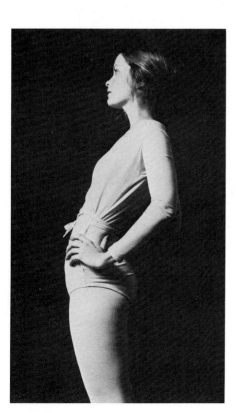

Lateral Walk

Helps develop balance and body coordination; helps promote strength in legs, ankles, and feet. From T'ai Chi.

1. Stand with feet 6 inches apart and parallel, knees slightly bent, with weight evenly distributed.
2. Slowly shift your weight onto right leg while moving left leg laterally left to a point on the ground where the leg is almost fully extended.
3. Slowly shift weight from right to left leg by bringing right foot to a point 6 inches from left and from original position.
4. Repeat steps 1, 2, and 3 three times. Your body will be traveling in a leftward direction. Shake the legs.
5. Repeat steps 1, 2, and 3 to the right side three times.

When moving laterally and shifting weight, keep eyes on the same horizontal line. You are continuously moving over distance. Your knees bend initially in step 1, lowering the level of eyes. Then eyes move on the smooth horizontal line, feet remaining parallel. Keep breathing into the spot below your navel.

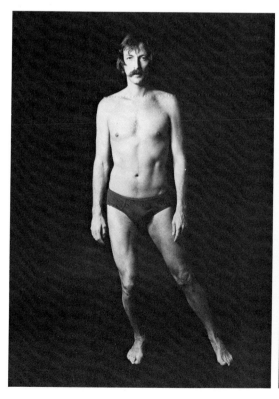 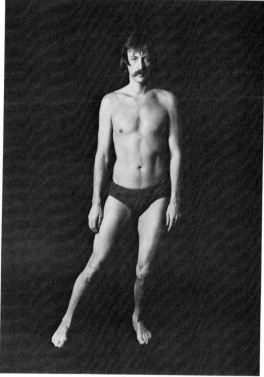

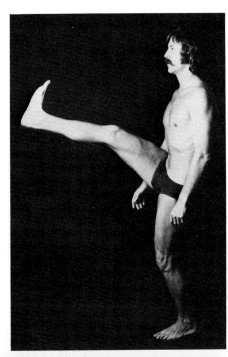

Jump Rope or Run in Place No. 3

Jump Rope: One-Legged Jump
(See page 55.) Increases endurance, cardiovascular and respiratory efficiency. Strengthens legs and feet. Improves grounding, coordination, and balance. From endurance training.

1 Jump Rope position.
2 Lift left foot from floor, jumping on right foot five times.
3 Change, lifting right foot from floor while jumping on left foot five times. Count to twenty; add twenty each week up to 100.
4 Continue jumping, but now on both feet, landing from balls of feet to heels 100 times. Add twenty-five per week up to 200. (That's 120 the first week—and 300 the fifth week—total for single leg and both legs.)

Shake out legs when finished; walk around room one minute, swinging arms. Do Integration Breath three times before you start next exercise. Monitor heart.

Run in Place No. 3
(See page 55.) Increases endurance, cardiovascular and respiratory efficiency. Strengthens legs, feet, arms, and shoulders. From endurance training.

Standing, raise each foot at least 6 inches off the floor to jog in place. Start with 400; add fifty per week until 550. After each 100 do ten jumping-jacks. Monitor heart rate. Rest 1 minute before you continue program. Walk and swing arms while breath returns to normal. Before next exercise do Integration Breath three times.

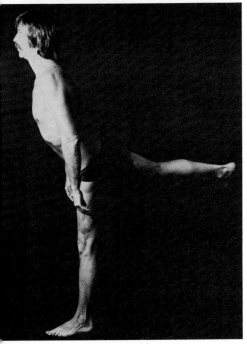

Pendulum Kick

Strengthens and stretches legs, develops balance. From Arica.

1 Standing, feet 6 inches apart, shift weight onto left leg until right leg is 1 inch from floor.
2 Kick straightened right leg forward up to waist level, with left knee slightly bent.
3 Return right leg toward floor; swing backward like a pendulum, keeping leg straight all the time. Do five kick-swings. Exhale when the leg is on the "up," inhaling on the "down."
4 Repeat with left leg.

Start with five kicks for each leg; add five each week until you reach twenty. When kicking forward, lead with the heel so that you feel the stretch throughout the leg. If you cannot kick waist high, kick as high as you can and work your way higher.

Masai Stand

Aids balance and grounding, strengthens legs. From yoga.

1 Standing, place right foot on inner left thigh, toes facing down.
2 Place palms together in front of chest; hold for a long deep breath into belly; then push hands together over head, arms close to ears.
3 Bring arms down, change to other leg.

Hold arms over head for four deep breaths; add two each week until you reach ten. Concentrate on an object somewhere in your line of vision. This will steady your body.

The Masai warriors stand for hours on one leg watching their herds. They do use their long spears to keep their balance, however.

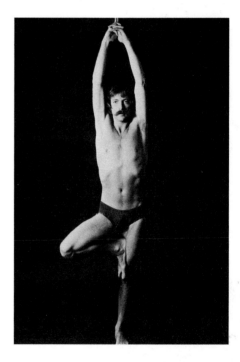

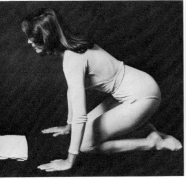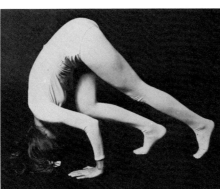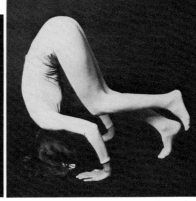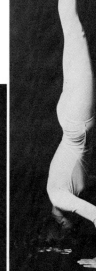

Head Stand

The flow of blood to the head nourishes brain, scalp, hair, complexion, vision, and hearing. Inverted body position stimulates organs and helps strengthen neck. This exercise should be done carefully and with caution. From yoga.

1 Sitting on heels, lean forward onto both hands, shoulder width apart.
2 Put top of your head between your hands, forming a triangle.
3 Walk slowly on toes to a vertical position causing trunk to be straight.
4 A gentle bounce will start feet and legs toward the sky; then elevate slowly until legs are straight.
5 Tuck knees into chest and slowly lower legs.

Before executing head stand, clear area of objects on which you could fall. Use a folded towel under head to prevent soreness.

Start with three deep breaths; add three per week up to twelve. This head stand can be practiced at first next to a wall for support, but learn not to rely on the wall.

Lion

Stretches root of tongue, face, and eye muscles. Stimulates throat. Improves skin and complexion. From yoga.

1 Rock pose, hands on knees.
2 Exhale a deep breath with a roar sound while opening throat, sticking your tongue out and down towards your chin. Eyes roll back as if looking over head. Fingers stretch apart, outward.

Do three times. Make sure throat is opened; closed, the sound can cause an irritation on the vocal cords. The lion can be done throughout the day in any of the sitting positions.

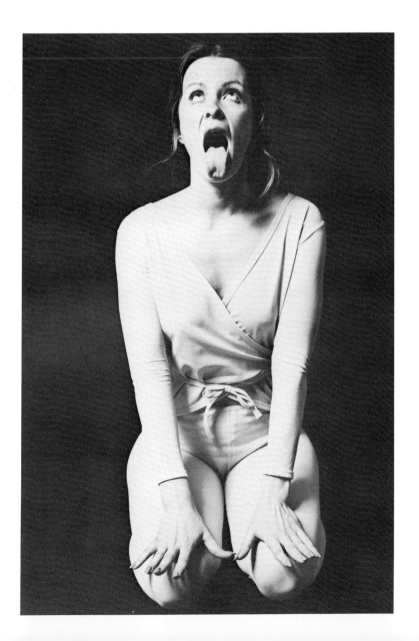

Contraction/Relaxation

Restores vitality. Done in Corpse Pose (see page 60).

1 Bring awareness to toes in your right foot; wiggle and stretch them. Spread toes apart. Relax.

2 Come up to ankle; rotate ankle, creating pressure.

3 Flex calf muscles. Relax.

4 Bring awareness to thigh. Tighten it, tighten it more. Lift your straightened leg off floor 2 inches, tighten more, then drop. Relax.

5 Roll your right leg. Become aware of left toes. Repeat technique for left leg.

6 From left thigh, take awareness to right hand. Rotate thumb and fingers; open and close palm. Stretch fingers and palm. Center of palm will rise slightly. Hold for one breath. Make a fist and rotate from wrist; create pressure for one breath. Straighten arm off floor 2 inches. Tighten fist, forearm, and upper arm as tight as you can for one breath and drop. Roll your leg.

7 Repeat with left hand and arm.

8 Contract muscles in rectum. If done correctly, your buttocks will rise from the ground. Tighten for one breath. Exhale and relax.

9 Breathe long and deep into belly. Holding breath for three counts, push out belly. Exhale rapidly through mouth.

10 After 10 seconds of normal breathing, expand chest. Push out from inside holding three counts; exhale rapidly through mouth.

11 Try to make shoulders meet over chest, holding for one breath; exhale and drop shoulders.

12 Move the muscles in your face, make ugly faces, big phony smiles to break down the tension. Imagine a paintbrush sticking out of your chin. Paint circles and figure eights on the ceiling and walls. Bring the energy into a small ball into the center of your face, trying to mash your lips against your nose. Inhale, exhale, releasing contractions in face.

13 Inhale long and deep into belly. Do not contract muscles. Imagine a white vibrational wave coming in through your toes and going out the top of your head. As you imagine this wave, be aware of the different parts of your body it passes on its journey up and out the top of your head.

Contract and tense muscles as tight as you can, release contraction and "let go" to achieve more relaxed state. Start from toes and think of each part of body until you reach head.

Chapter 9

Cycle IV

Warm-Up:

Cleansing Breath
Roll in Ball

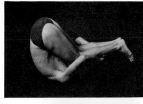

Sky/Earth Picking Apples/Hip-Up

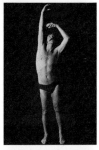

Camel Neck Roll

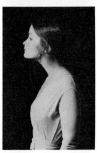

Exercises:

Shoulder Roll/
Waist Bend

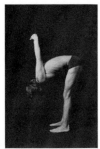

Forward Stretch/
Foot on Thigh

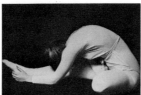

Knee to
Chest/
Kick-
Out

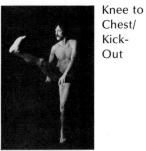

Leg Swing

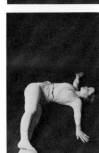

Wrist Circles
(Rock Pose)

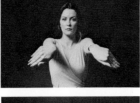

Archer

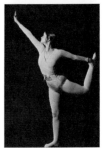

Pullup or Reverse
Pushup

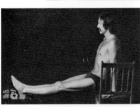

Pelvic Bounce/
Arch-Up

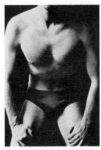

Head Star

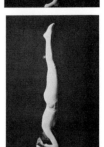

Top Twist

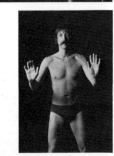

Abdominal
Pump

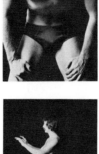

Eye Exerci

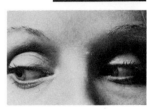

Pelvic Rotation
Push Air

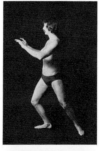

Contracti
Relaxatio

Leg Scissors

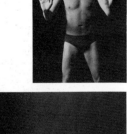

Opposite Arm/Leg
Raise

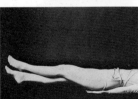

Body Swings

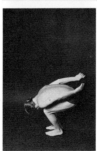

Cleansing Breath

Stimulates and purifies lungs and tones respiratory organs. Mainly used after other breathing exercises as a refresher.

1   Inhale complete breath.
2   Retain.
3   Purse lips as if to whistle, but do not puff out cheeks.
4   Exhale a little air vigorously by quickly pulling and contracting abdominal muscles—then hold. Continue little by little, with vigor, until you have exhaled completely.

Do three breaths.

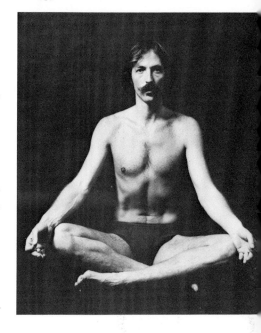

Roll in Ball

Stretches and stimulates spine. Good warm-up. From Kundalini.

1   Sitting, hold knees up against chest with arms.
2   Still holding knees to chest, push off heels backwards, rolling length of spine toward head.
3   With a downward motion against legs, push off from back to original position.

Start with ten; add five each week up to twenty-five. Eventually you will be able to roll to standing position when ready for the next posture.

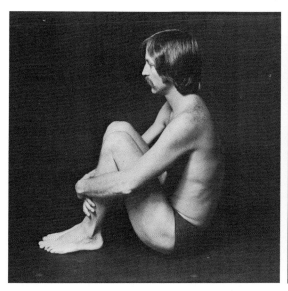

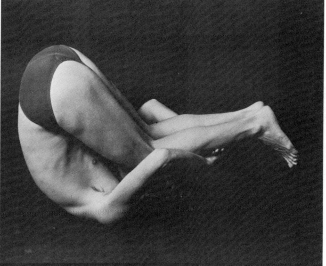

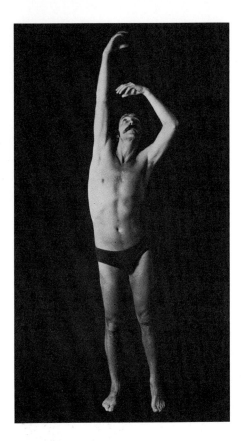

Sky/Earth Picking Apples/Hip-Up

Benefits body in same way as Sky/Earth Picking Apples, adding extra stretch to sides of torso.

1 Standing, feet at shoulder width and parallel, inhale reaching arms up toward the sky.
2 Exhale and slowly bring arms down to sides. Repeat once.
3 Inhale, arms up, reaching for imaginary apple with right hand; lift left hip and heel from floor. Keep toes on floor.
4 When reaching for the apple with the left hand, lift right hip up and lift heel from floor.
5 Exhale, dropping arms and bending from waist; lightly bounce hands, arms, and shoulders toward floor three times. When bending from waist, touch hand to floor behind heels.
6 Inhale and stretch toward sky picking apples, repeating Items 3 and 4.

Alternate reaching for apple three times before bending from waist. Reach—and think—higher and higher.

While bending, legs are kept straight.

Camel Neck Roll

Helps relieve headache, stimulates thyroid gland and cervical section of spine. Firms chin and neck.

1 Standing with feet 6 inches apart, move your chin forward and tuck in toward neck.
2 Tuck chin into chest; then bring chin up, facing forward, tilting head back, up and forward into original position.

Start with four in each direction listed in instruction # 2; add two each week until you reach ten. The head moves similarly to a person's head when riding a camel.

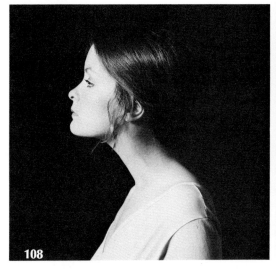
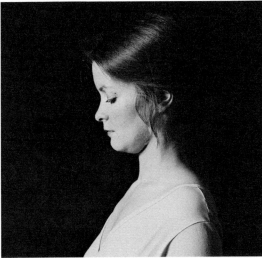

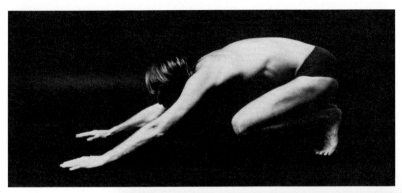

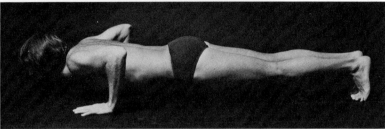

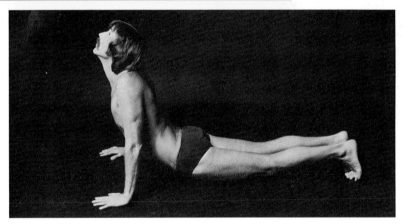

Salute to the Sun/Dip

Variation of Salute to the Sun. Gives strength to arms.

1   From the body in the pushup position (step 5 in Salute to the Sun [p. 47]), move backward to a squatting position, knees close to chest.
2   Dip arms at elbows, move chest forward and parallel to the floor a few inches above it, pushing from feet.
3   When legs are extended, move head and shoulders up into a Cobra position without your body touching the floor.
4   Continue into regular step 8 position of Salute to the Sun.

Do three times.

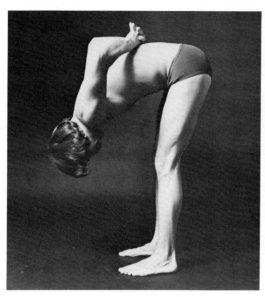
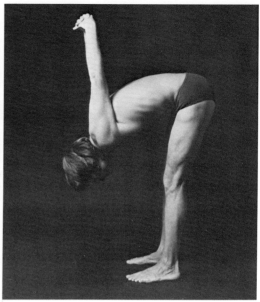

Shoulder Roll/Waist Bend

Stretches shoulders and spine. Helps relieve back pain. From Arica.

1　Standing erect, feet 6 inches apart and parallel, clasp hands together behind buttocks.
2　Exhale, bending forward at waist while moving hands up along spinal column.
3　Inhale, pushing hands toward sky in a forward direction.
4　Still inhaling, raise body up from waist stretching shoulders back and into original position.

Start with four; add two each week until you reach ten. The movement is a continuous motion.

Leg Swing

Tones abdominal muscles, stretches joints in spinal column. From isotonics.

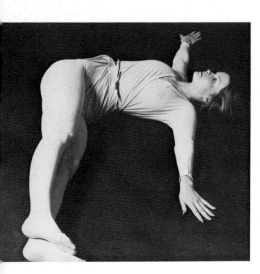

1　Lie on your back, arms out to the sides, palms down in a perpendicular plane, legs extended up toward sky.
2　Exhaling, swing legs to the right side touching floor. (Keep knees straight.) Leg movement is continuous.
3　Inhale, swinging legs back up past center; exhale down to left.
4　Inhale, legs back to center.

Start with five swings on each side; add five per week until you reach twenty. Keep legs together, shoulders and head on floor.

Pullup or Reverse Pushup

Pullup

Strengthens arms, chest and shoulder muscles. From isotonics.

1 Hold onto horizontal bar, palms facing away from you.
2 Inhale while pulling yourself up until chin is even with bar. Slowly come back to original hanging position while exhaling.

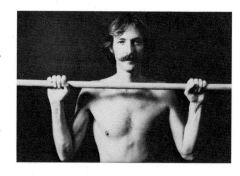

Do two pullups, rest, and, breathing normally, do two more. Add one weekly to reach five and five. If two is too many, try one and build. You can only get stronger. The horizontal bar can be a water pipe, tree limb, or door molding. Make sure it's secure before putting all your weight on it. If you do not have access to a bar, do the alternate exercise, Reverse Pushup.

Reverse Pushup

Strengthens arms and shoulders. From isotonics.

1 Resting on your palms and heels, each palm on a chair, feet together on a lower footrest or other support, legs straight, exhale, bend arms, lowering your body down between chairs.
2 Inhale. Return to step 1 position.

Start with five; add five each week until you reach twenty. Chairs on which palms are resting should be placed slightly further apart than shoulders.

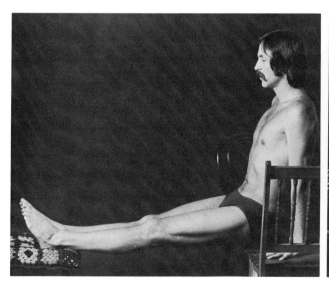 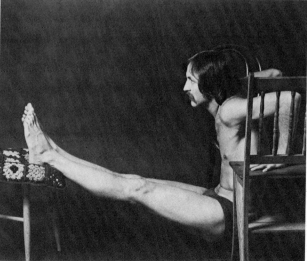

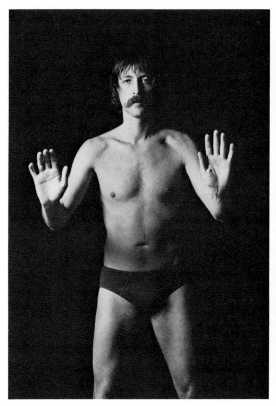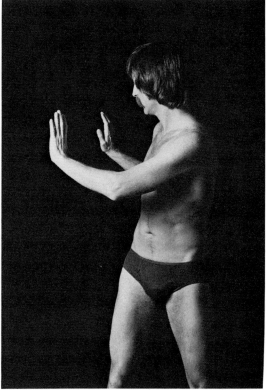

Top Twist

Strengthens legs, helps grounding, stretches pelvis, and tones side waist muscles. From Kung Fu.

1 Stand with feet slightly wider than shoulders, legs slightly bent at knees, arms in front, slightly bent at elbows, hands in a position as if ready to hold a wall from collasping, placed almost at shoulder height.
2 Inhale, twist head, arms, and shoulders to the right, keeping pelvis area to the front.
3 Exhale while swinging forward.
4 Inhale turning to the left, keeping pelvis front.
5. Exhale while swinging forward.

Start with ten; add ten each week until you reach forty.

So pelvis will not swing around with shoulders when twisting right, think of pelvis turning left; when twisting left, think of pelvis turning right. Coordinate the breath movement so there is no hesitation in torso when swinging forward. Remember to turn head.

Leg Scissors

Tones abdominal muscles, gives strength to lower back. Stimulates abdominal organs. Isotonic.

1 Lie on your back, hands and fingers underneath lower buttocks, palms down.

2 Lift legs off floor 6 inches, alternate crossing right ankle over left, left over right in a scissor motion. At start repeat ten times. Return to floor. Rest on a count of ten.

3 Lift legs one foot off floor widening the scissors to cross at the knee. Do ten times. Return to floor. Rest on a count of ten.

4 Lift legs 18 inches off floor, widening the scissors to cross at the upper thigh. Do ten times.

Start with ten crosses, counting one each time right leg is on top. Increase five each week until you reach twenty-five. Movement is continuous.

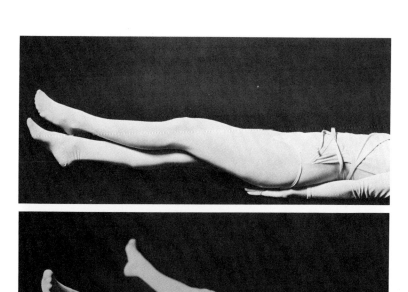

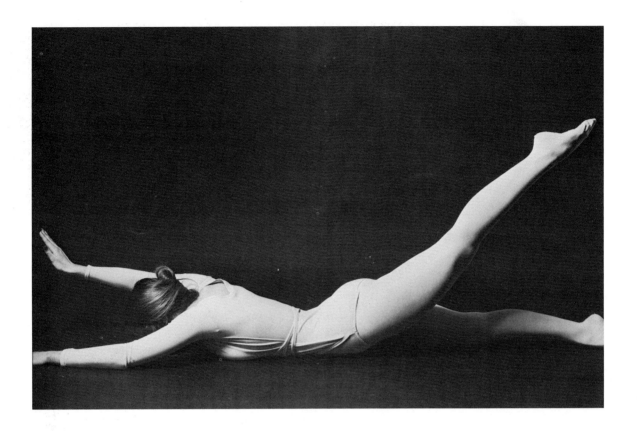

Opposite Arm/Leg Raise

Helps digestion, coordination, relieves constipation. Strengthens back muscles. From yoga.

1 Lie on stomach, arms extended on ground over head, palms down, feet together.
2 Inhale, raising right arm from shoulder and left leg from hip. Retain breath for three counts.
3 Exhale, lowering arm and leg slowly to floor.
4 Inhale, raising left arm and right leg. Retain breath for three counts.
5 Exhale, lowering arm and leg slowly to floor.

Start with five extensions on each side; add one per week until you reach ten. Lift arms, legs, and head as high as possible. Then try this without lifting head off floor.

Forward Stretch/Foot on Thigh

Includes benefits of forward stretch, plus additional stretching of inner thigh and buttocks. From Kundalini.

1 Sit on floor, legs extended.
2 Bend right knee, placing right foot on top of left thigh. Gently bounce right knee toward floor a few times.
3 Inhale, stretch arms and torso toward sky.
4 Exhale, bending forward, holding onto the farthest part of leg your hands come in contact with. (Ultimately you will hold toes, with your head to your knees.)
5 Relax head between shoulders; close eyes and breathe long and deep ten breaths.
6 Inhale while coming up slowly.
7 Change legs and repeat.

Start with ten long deep breaths; add five each week up to twenty-five. Take a few seconds to lightly bounce knees, and go into Corpse Pose.

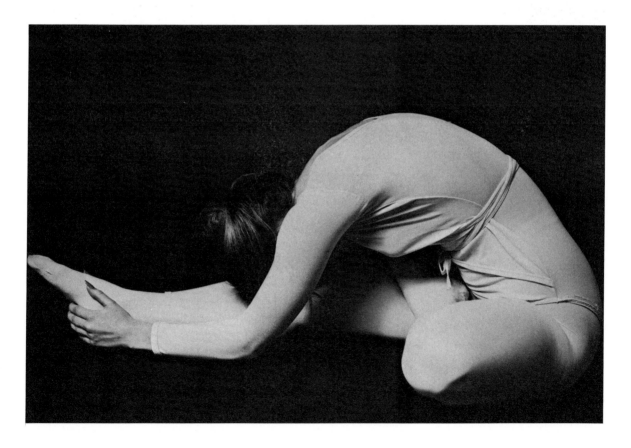

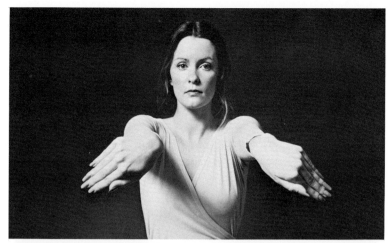

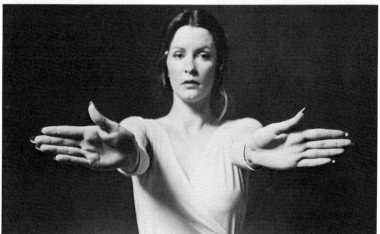

Wrist Circles (Rock Pose)

Stimulates and strengthens wrists, forearms, and shoulders while stretching thighs and ankles. Develops poise and grace in arms and hands. From Arica.

1　Sitting in Rock Pose, raise arms to horizontal position, elbows slightly bent, palms facing each other.
2　Circle hands, palms out, from wrist five times toward the inside—right hand moving counterclockwise, left hand clockwise—while inhaling.
3　Circle hands from wrist five times toward the outside (right hand moving clockwise, left hand counterclockwise). Exhale five times.

This is one round. Start with four rounds, add two rounds each week up to ten. Feel the pressure on your wrists. Breathe into the belly.

Pelvic Bounce/Arch-Up

(See Pelvic Bounce, page 97.) Helps energy flow into pelvic area. Helps open pelvic blocks. Stretches and strengthens lower back.

1   Do pelvic bounce thirty times. (See page 97.)
2   Inhale, raising pelvis to sky.
3   Exhale, returning pelvis to original position.

Start with six; add two each week up to ten.

Breathe through mouth into belly.

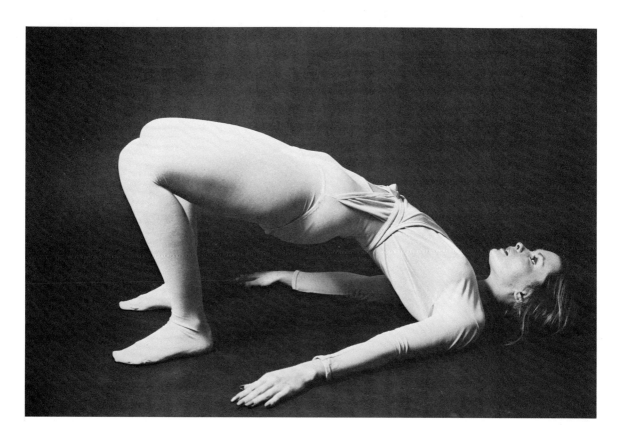

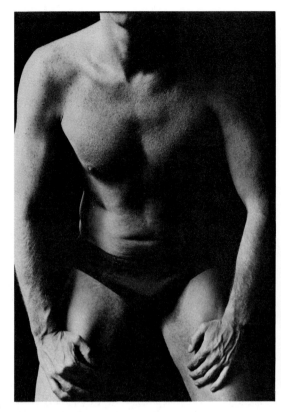 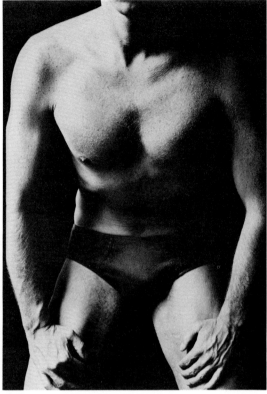

Abdominal Pump

Stimulates and massages abdominal organs, relieves indigestion, constipation, and liver problems while toning abdominal muscles and increasing circulation. A yoga technique.

1   Standing, feet at shoulder width, bend trunk forward, placing hands on thighs.
2   Empty lungs of air with a deep exhalation while contracting abdominal muscles. Imagine touching your navel to your spinal column.
3   While locking the breath out, pump abdominal muscles forward (making a pot belly) and then back to original hollow position. This is one pump. Start with ten pumps. This is one round. Rest 15 seconds. Do two rounds. Add five pumps each week until you reach twenty-five.

Pelvic Rotation

Helps flexibility and loosens pelvic tension. Strengthens lower back. A bioenergetics technique.

1 Lying on your back, feet as near buttocks as possible, arms on floor, raise pelvis.
2 Rotate pelvis in a clockwise circular motion for five revolutions.
3 Change direction to counterclockwise for five revolutions.

Start with five in each direction; add five per week until you reach twenty. When beginning, placing palms on the floor will help balance. Breathe through mouth into belly.

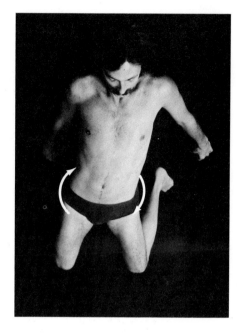

Push Air

Increases mobility in ankles, knees, and thighs. Helps coordination and balance, and helps the body to move as a unit. Based on T'ai Chi.

1 Stand with feet parallel and slightly wider than shoulders, knees slightly bent.
2 Shift weight onto left leg, bending left knee deeper while right heel pivots and right foot is perpendicular to left.
3 With right leg straight, foot flat on floor, and shoulders and hips facing direction of right foot, lift hands to chest level.
4 Push air with hands toward right foot. As you push off from left leg, feel the weight shift to both legs, then onto right leg, which becomes bent, left leg straight.
5 Shift weight back onto left leg. Push air three times.
6 Change to right side three times.
Three times on each side is one round.

Start with three rounds; add one each week, until you reach six rounds. Try to bend knees lower and twist hips and shoulders in direction of pivot foot.

While pushing air, there is a feeling of pushing an automobile—but without strength or tension. Body moves as a whole. Breathe into belly. Be aware of the point three fingers below navel. Movements are performed slowly.

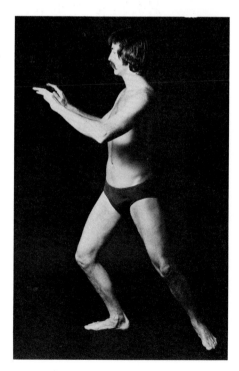

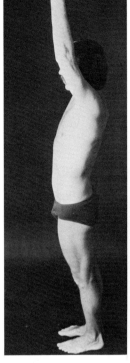
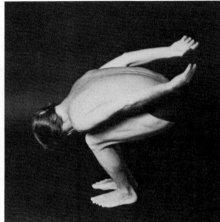

Body Swings

Overall body stretch. Strengthens leg muscles, helps grounding. Increases cardiovascular and respiratory efficiency. An American Mime Theater exercise.

1   Stand with feet 6 inches apart, arms overhead, palms facing each other.
2   Exhale, swing arms straight down while bending forward and squatting, heels and toes in contact with floor. Follow through to rear.
3   Inhale and swing arms back to original standing position.

Start with twenty; add ten each week until you reach fifty swings.

The arm swings start the movement down, and the torso follows a moment later—likewise when standing, similar to a racing dive into the sky.

Monitor heart rate. Rest 1 minute before continuing. Do three Integration Breaths.

Knee to Chest/Kick-Out

Helps bring energy flow to pelvis, stretches and strengthens legs, helps in balance and grounding. From Kung Fu.

1   Standing with feet 6 inches apart, lift right knee toward chest, kick right leg straight out while exhaling in one fluid motion. Lower leg.

2   Repeat five kicks.

3   Repeat, using left leg.

4   Repeat five kicks. This is one round.

Start with two rounds; add one each week until you reach five. Make them explosive, quick kicks. Assist with hands if necessary in order to bring knee up toward chest.

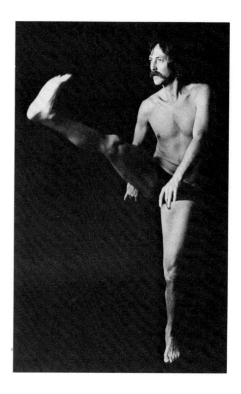

Archer

Develops balance and poise. Stretches and strengthens lower back and thigh muscles. From yoga.

1   Standing, hold right ankle with right hand.

2   Raise left hand to a slight angle forward and above shoulder while lifting right leg to a slight angle to right. Concentrate on your fingertips.

3   Change to other leg.

Balance for four deep breaths; add two breaths each week until you reach ten.

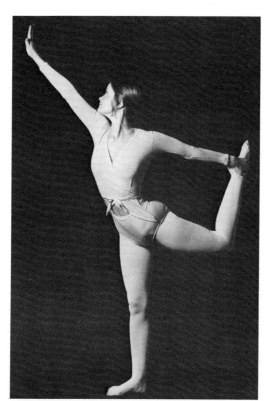

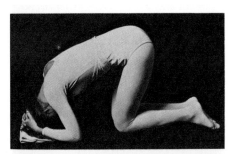
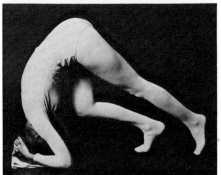
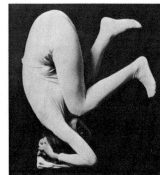
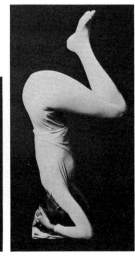
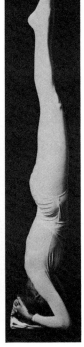

Head Stand

Increases supply of blood carrying oxygen to the brain, eyes, and ears. Helps relieve and prevent varicose veins. Stimulates circulation in scalp. This exercise should be done carefully and with caution. From yoga.

Use a folded towel under head to prevent soreness. Remember that the exact placement of elbows will determine your ability to stay balanced in the posture. If your elbows are too far apart, chances are you will fall either forward or backward; if too close together, the fall will be to the side. When forming triangle between elbows and hands, touch fingers of right hand to inside of left elbow. Then pivot right arm on right elbow to interlock fingers.

1 Sitting on knees, form a tripod by interlocking fingers and both elbows as a base on floor in front of you.
2 Place the top of your head on the floor, hands supporting back of head.

3 Walk forward on toes, raising your torso into an almost vertical position, knees close to body.

4 Push up lightly, slowly raising legs into the air until the body is vertical.

5 Bring knees into chest, lower legs slowly.

Start with three deep breaths in posture; add five each week until you reach eighteen. Before executing head stand, clear area of objects on which you could fall.

The head stand is one of the most powerful postures in yoga.

Eye Exercise
Stretches and promotes circulation for eye muscles, relief for tired eyes.

1 Sitting in Easy Pose, move eyes as directed.

2 Horizontal: right to left, left to right.

3 Vertical: up and down.

4 Diagonal: upper right to lower left and back.

5 Diagonal: upper left to lower right and back.

6 Letter "U": upper right swing down and up to upper left—and back.

7 Describe a rainbow: lower right swing up and down to lower left—and back.

8 Rub palms together, generating heat. Place palms on eyes for 5 seconds.

9 Lightly stroke eyelids from side to side with fingertips (do this twice).

Do each eye movement three times, stretching to the extremes but not straining. Close eyes a moment between each exercise. Do not move the head.

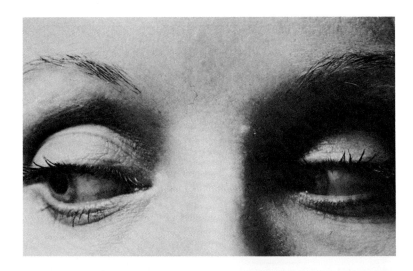

Contraction/Relaxation

Restores vitality. Do this one in the Corpse Pose.

1   Bring awareness to toes in your right foot, wiggle them and stretch them. Spread toes apart. Relax.

2   Come up to ankle; rotate ankle, creating pressure.

3   Flex calf muscles. Relax.

4   Bring awareness to thigh. Tighten it, tighten it more. Lift straightened leg off floor 2″, tighten more, then drop. Relax.

5   Roll your right leg. Become aware of left toes. Repeat technique for left leg.

6   From left thigh, take awareness to right hand. Rotate thumb and fingers, open and close palm. Stretch fingers and palm. Center of palm will rise slightly. Hold for one breath. Make a fist and rotate from wrist; create pressure for one breath. Straighten arm off floor 2 inches. Tighten fist, forearm, and upper arm as tight as you can for one breath and drop. Roll.

7   Repeat with left hand and arm.

8   Contract muscles in rectum. If done correctly, your buttocks will rise from the ground. Tighten for one breath. Exhale and relax.

9   Breathe long and deep into belly. Holding breath for three counts, push out belly. Exhale rapidly through mouth.

10 After 10 seconds of normal breathing, expand chest. Push out from inside holding three counts; exhale rapidly through mouth.

11 Try to make shoulders meet over chest, holding for one breath; exhale and drop shoulders.

12 Move the muscles in your face, make ugly faces, big phony smiles to break down the tension. Imagine a paintbrush sticking out of your chin. Paint circles and figure eights on the ceiling and walls. Bring the energy into a small ball into the center of your face trying to mash your lips against your nose. Inhale, exhale, releasing contractions in face.

13 Inhale long and deep into belly. Do not contract muscles. Imagine a white vibrational wave coming in through your toes and going out the top of your head. As you imagine this wave, be aware of the different parts of your body it passes on its journey up and out the top of your head.

Contract and tense muscles as tight as you can, then release contraction and "let go" to achieve a more relaxed state. Start from your toes and think of each part of the body until you reach your head.

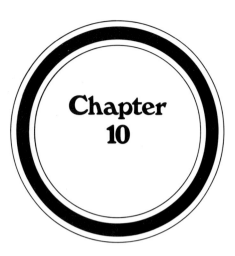

Chapter 10

Cycle V

Warm-Up:

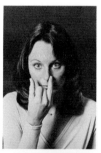

Alternate Breathing

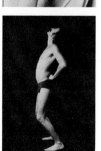

Bioenergetic Bend

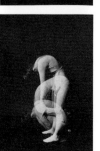

The Stretch

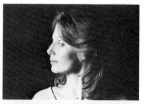

Look Left/Turn Right

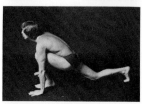

The Sprinter

Exercises:

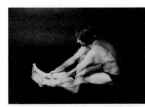
Forward Stretch Wha Guru

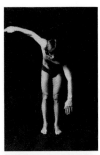
Swimmer

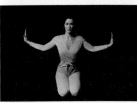
Pull Back Fingers (Rock Pose)

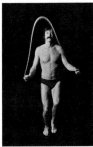
Jump Rope (Speed)/Run in Place No. 4

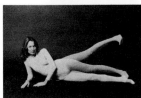
Empty Saddle Bags

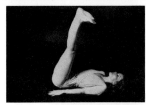
Pelvic Bounce/ Arch/ Leg Raise

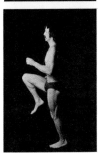

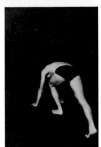
Pushup/ Hand Stand

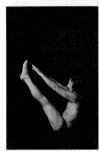
Jackknife

Front Roundho Kick

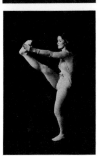

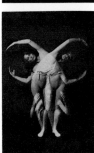
Squat Lateral/Ball

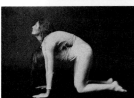
Cat and Cow

Skate
Shoulder Stand Plough

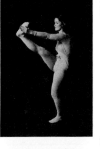

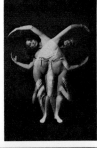
Leg Circles

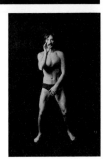
Coordination

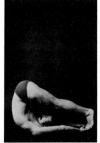

Bridge to Whee

Contraction/ Relaxation

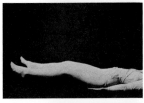
The Sail

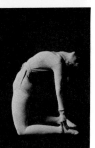

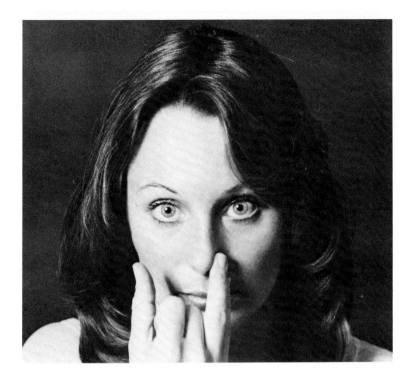

Alternate Breathing
Calms nerves, prevents insomnia.

1 Sit cross-legged; tuck index and middle finger into base of thumb (lower fatty part) in palm of right hand.
2 Close right nostril with thumb; exhale steadily through left nostril.
3 At the end of exhalation, inhale through left nostril deeply and slowly.
4 At the end of inhalation, open right nostril and close left nostril with ring finger and pinky, exhaling steadily through right nostril.
5 At the end of exhalation, inhale through right nostril.
6 Depress right nostril with thumb and continue cycle without holding breath.

Do 1 minute and increase as you become comfortable.

This exercise is good to do at night if you have trouble sleeping. After several weeks of practicing alternate breathing, you may start doubling your exhalation count. For example, go from eight inhalations to sixteen exhalations, increasing the number of rounds.

When you can maintain fifty rounds comfortably, begin holding breath between inhalation and exhalation, a ratio of 1-4-2. (E.g., inhale 4, hold 16, exhale 8.) Holding may be done by depressing both nostrils.

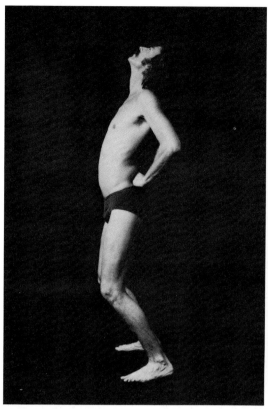

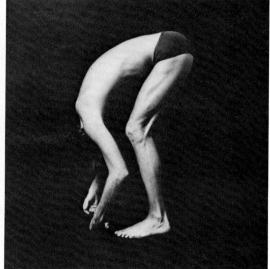

Bioenergetic Bend

A warm-up to get your energy flowing. Helps grounding.

1 Stand, feet at shoulder width, toes slightly turned inward.
2 Place fists on small of your back and lean back. Breathe into belly.
3 Move your head backward, which will arch your back more. Stay in this position for at least 1 minute.
4 Lean forward, round back, head relaxed, arms dangling, fingers touching floor. Stay in this position for at least 1 minute.

You may experience vibrations in your legs. Just let them shake, you are using your muscles in a new and different way.

The Stretch

Overall body stretch. Strengthens legs, aids in grounding. From the American Mime Theater.

1 Stand, feet 6 inches apart, slowly rotate head forward, chin to chest.
2 Shoulders and upper back rotate forward.
3 Bend trunk forward from waist.
4 When shoulders reach waist level, start bending at knees, bringing arms behind legs and moving into a squat (See first photograph.)
5 Clasp wrist in back of ankles, unbending knees to straighten legs (See second photograph.)
6 Squat again, drop wrist, and slowly stand, straightening up trunk, shoulders, back, and head.

Do three, move slowly vertebra by vertebra.

Breathe long and deep while doing this exercise.

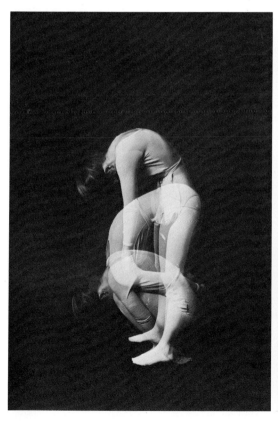
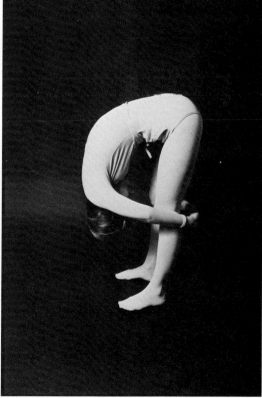

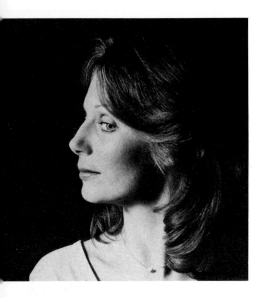

Look Left/Turn Right

Breaks down neck patterns and habits. Helps coordination, relieves headaches. From Chinese medicine.

1 Stand, feet 6 inches apart.
2 Turn head to the right as eyes look left.
3 Turn head to the left as eyes look right.

Start with four turns to each side; add two per week until you reach ten.

Try to catch something to look at out of the corner of your eye to stretch muscles.

The Sprinter

Stretches spine and legs. Helps strengthen arms, shoulders, lower back, and legs.

1 Squat with feet 1 foot apart, hands on floor, fingers facing forward.
2 Extend right leg back to rear, knee touching floor.
3 Then, in one bouncing movement, extend left leg to the rear, bringing right leg to the front, reversing the position of feet.

Each time right leg is forward counts one. Start with ten; add five each week until you reach twenty-five. The closer your feet get to your hands, the more stretch your legs feel. Try this one on your fingertips.

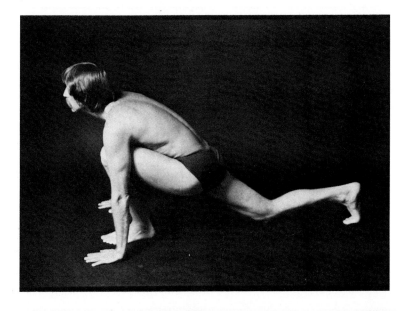

Swimmer

Stretches and conditions shoulders and upper back. Helps coordination and swimming technique.

1 Standing erect, feet 6 inches apart and parallel, raise right arm, fingers toward sky and palm facing forward, left arm down, palm facing behind you.
2 Right arm moves down forward as left arm moves back and up.
3 Continue stroking arms in circles as if swimming. Do thirty strokes freestyle (forward).
4 Reverse direction of stroke. Do thirty strokes backstroke.
5 Bend at waist (see photo). Do thirty strokes freestyle.

Start with thirty strokes; add ten each week until you reach sixty.

Move the arms at different speeds, staying aware of centering. When stroking from waist-bend position, throw arm forward. It's like flipping the arm forward almost out of control, but that's the time when the muscles can relax. Find that moment (without tension) and discover one of the keys to endurance.

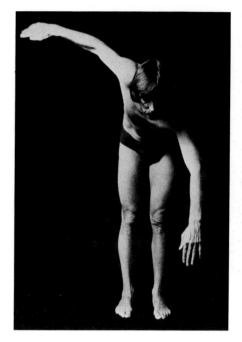

Empty Saddle Bags

Tones flabby outer thighs.

1 Lie on right side, right elbow, forearm, and left hand for support, both legs straight.
2 Flex left foot, point toes toward head, foot parallel to floor.
3 Keeping left leg straight, inhale and raise it as high as possible.
4 Exhale, lowering left leg on top of right leg.
5 Repeat on left side, with right leg.

Lift each leg ten times, add ten lifts each leg per week until you reach thirty. Keep the angle of your pelvis perpendicular to floor and your hips rolled forward—there is a tendency to roll back. Variation: To make the hip muscle work harder, increase the angle of head and shoulders from floor. Move up from elbow to hand on the floor, gradually extending arm.

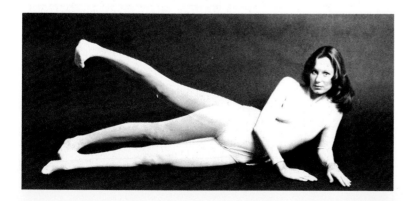

Pushup/Hand Stand

Strengthens shoulders, arms, and wrists; develops balance; stimulates internal organs. This exercise should be done carefully and with caution. An isotonic exercise.

1 Place hands on floor at shoulder width, 6 inches from a solid wall.
2 Head down, walk two or three small steps toward the wall.
3 Push off from both feet with enough kick to get legs toward the sky. Feet should then touch and balance against wall.
4 Do two pushups, bending elbows and lowering your body down as far as strength allows.
5 Tuck in waist, knees to chest, coming down to floor.

Start with two; add one a week until you reach seven. When you kick legs against wall, arch back to help get your feet in the direction of wall. At first lower your body 1 or 2 inches; build to get lower, adding repetitions. Do not try to get chin to floor the first month.

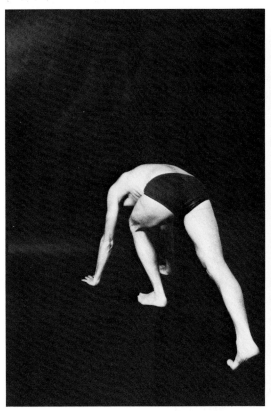
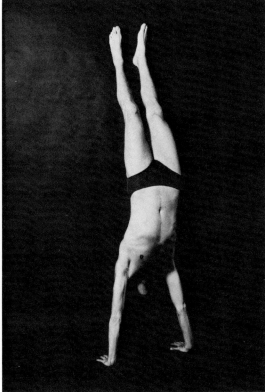

Squat Lateral/Ball

Helps tone side abdominal muscles, which are often neglected in exercise. Strengthens foot, leg, thigh, and lower back muscles and aids peristalsis. The flat-footed squat helps in grounding. From Arica.

1 Stand, feet 6 inches to 12 inches apart, and bend knees into a squat position while exhaling. Try to keep the entire bottoms of your feet on the ground.

2 Inhale as you push down against the ground with the full foot as you return to a standing position.

3 As you get to the top, throw your right arm over your head, left hand out to the left side. Try to feel as if you are holding a ball between your hands.

4 Repeat with the other side.

Start with twenty squats on each side; add ten each week until you reach fifty. Go through the motion slowly while learning, then increase to any speed and rhythm that works for you. Music can set the pace.

Keeping the feet flat on the ground during step 1 is difficult for many people—athletic or not—so don't be discouraged. Your muscles will stretch and relax to the point where you will see improvement after a few sessions.

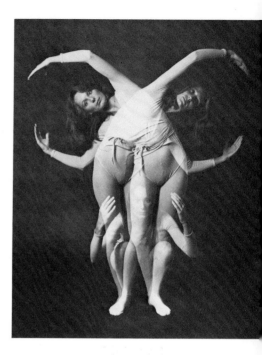

Leg Circles

Tones abdominal muscles, gives strength to lower back. Isotonic.

1 Lie on your back, hands and fingers underneath lower buttocks, palms down.

2 Lift legs off floor 6 inches, knees slightly flexed. Describe small circles simultaneously with each leg—ten circles one way, then ten circles the other. Lower legs.

3 Rest.

4 Lift legs 18 inches; repeat circles, making them larger—ten one way, ten the other. Lower legs.

5 Rest.

6 Lift legs 3 feet; repeat circles, making them larger—ten one way, ten the other. Lower legs.

Start with ten; add five each week until you reach twenty-five. Breathe into belly.

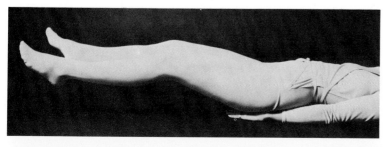

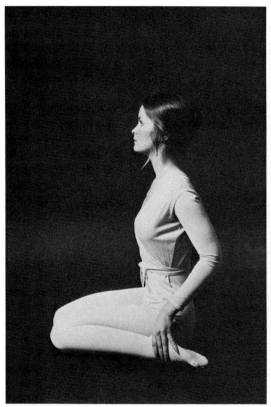
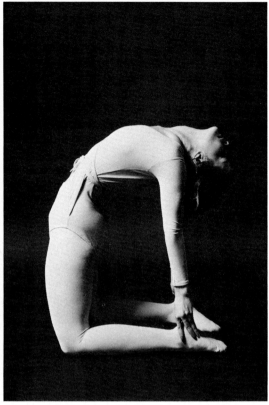

The Sail

Good overall stretch for lower and upper back, neck, thighs, and ankles. Helps energy flow, opening pelvis blocks. Adds strength to arms. From Kundalini.

1 Sit in Rock Pose with knees and feet open; sit between heels.
2 Grasp heels, inhale, raising pelvis forward and up, head slowly dropping back, arms extended, elbows straightened. (If you are not yet flexible enough to raise pelvis, sit up and slowly lean back to grasp heels.)
3 In this position do Breath of Fire. Imagine your exhalation is the wind beating forward your pelvic area—the Sail.
4 Exhale, sitting.

Start with thirty Breaths of Fire; add ten each week until you reach seventy.

Forward Stretch Wha Guru

Spine becomes elastic and muscles in back of legs are stretched; nerves are stimulated. Kundalini.

1 Sit on floor, legs extended together in front.
2 Inhale, stretch arms and torso toward sky.
3 Exhale, bending forward to grasp ankles.
4 Inhale, raising head, then bend elbows and exhale forward and down.
5 Using Breath of Fire rhythm, inhale up extending arms, elbows straight, exhale forward and down bending elbows.
6 When finished repetitions exhale down, hold for a count, then inhale up and lie back into Corpse Pose.

Start with forty Breaths of Fire; add twenty each week until you reach 100. Be careful not to hit your head on your knee. Keep legs straight, toes pointed upward. Imagine you are pulling through your heels. The name Wha Guru originated from its effect upon the practitioner. After executing it for 31 minutes—"Wow, guru!"

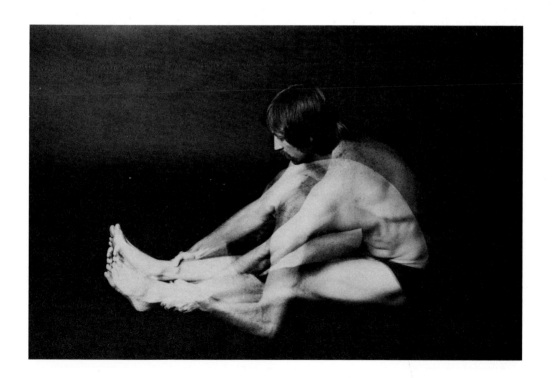

Pull Back Fingers (Rock Pose)

Stimulates and strengthens wrists, forearms, and fingers. Develops grace and flexibility in wrists and fingers. From Kung Fu.

1   Sitting in Rock Pose, extend arms, elbows slightly bent, out horizontally to the sides, palms vertical as if you were holding back a wall from closing in on you.
2   From the wrist, pull fingers and back of hand back toward your head.
3   Return to imaginary wall.

Start with fifteen; add five each week until you reach thirty. Breathe into belly.

The second part of this exercise releases and relaxes any tension caused by the first.

1   Sitting in the same position—the Rock Pose—imagine 5-pound-weight pulleys on the imaginary wall.
2   Open your hand, slowly grasp imaginary horizontal handles, and pull toward shoulders, releasing over shoulders.

Release and retrieve imaginary pulley five to ten times. Five pounds is quite light, so a minimum of imaginary tension should be created.

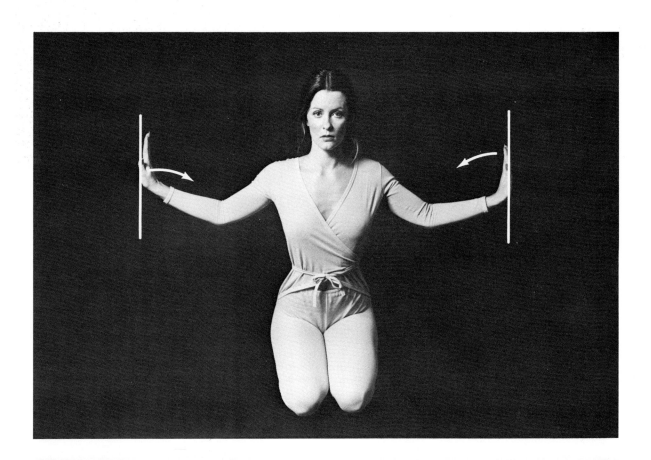

Pelvic Bounce/Arch/Leg Raise

Helps energy flow into pelvic area. Stretches lower back and back of legs. Strengthens lower back.

1 Do pelvic bounce thirty times (see page 97).
2 Do pelvic arch-up ten times (see page 117).
3 Bring sacrum* back to floor; extend legs to sky, toes pointing toward head and downward for maximum stretch.

Start with ten long, deep breaths; add two each week up to sixteen.

Try to push your heels to the sky. To get a better idea of what that feels like, reach up and pull your toes toward your head. You will probably roll back. Try to straighten legs, holding toes. When you let go of your toes you will roll back onto the sacrum. Your legs may vibrate—but that's fine, because it's your energy you're feeling. Breathe through your mouth into your belly.

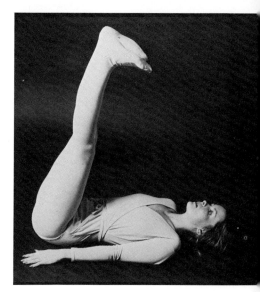

Jackknife

Tones abdomen, thigh, and lower back muscles; develops balance. From yoga.

1 Lie on your back, arms extended on floor over shoulders.
2 Jackknife legs, torso, and arms up, hands touching toes, balancing on sacrum. Return to floor.

Start with ten; add three each week up to twenty. Balance on sacrum. Touch toes for one count. Exhale up—inhale down.

*Sacrum: the place between the buttocks and small of back.

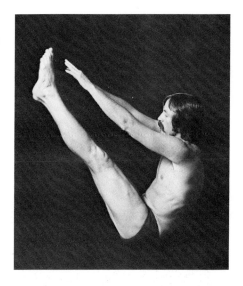

Cat and Cow

Develops pelvic control, endurance, and coordination, allowing movement in a combination of different ways. Relieves lower back pain. Releases pelvic blocks.

1 Position yourself on your hands and knees, knees shoulder width apart.

2 Tilt head back. Curve back downward, slightly lower than buttocks, in swayback position.

3 Exhale, while dropping your head low enough to look through your legs, simultaneously thrusting your pelvis forward and arching your back like a frightened cat.

4 Inhale, tilting head backward to original position while dropping your back into swayback position and rotating pelvis.

Imagine your head and buttocks are on hinges; they move up and down together in two clean movements. Start slowly while learning the motion. Increase speed and rhythm to fire breathing (count each exhalation as one breath). Begin with twenty breaths; add ten each week until you reach fifty.

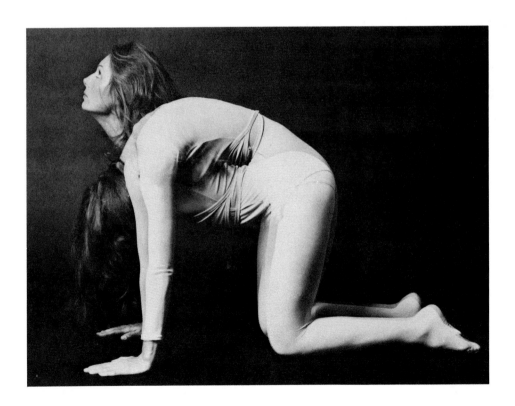

Coordination

Develops coordination and graceful arms. Good for self-defense. From Kung Fu.

1. Standing, feet parallel, wider than shoulder width, knees slightly bent. Right hand in front of throat, palm facing outward, pointing down; left hand is in front of groin, palm facing in.
2. Slowly, right hand traces a clockwise circle while left hand simultaneously traces a counterclockwise circle in the same vertical plane. Neither hand crosses the other's path.
3. Continue moving arms, slowly increasing the speed until you are flinging your arms effortlessly.

Start with 30 seconds; increase to 1 minute. Concentrate first on your hands, finding the exact line of flight. Move your awareness of the motion to your elbows, then to your shoulders. Finally, forget your arm and center your attention three fingers below your navel. Breathe into that place. (The circle traces overlap, but hands do not hit because when one hand in on top, the other is at the bottom.)

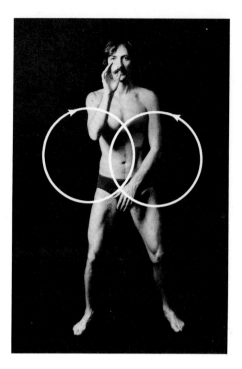

Jump Rope (Speed)/Run in Place No. 4

Jump Rope (Speed)

(See page 55.) Increases endurance, cardiovascular and respiratory efficiency. Strengthens legs and feet. Improves balance, grounding, and coordination. From endurance training.

1. Jump Rope position.
2. Jump off both feet, landing on balls of feet with knees slightly bent, then softly touching heels to floor.

Start with 300; add fifty each week until you reach 500. Breathe through mouth. Remember to do Integration Breath before next exercise. Monitor heart rate.

Run in Place No. 4

Increases endurance, cardiovascular and respiratory efficiency. Strengthens legs, feet, arms, and shoulders. From endurance training.

Standing, raise each foot, in turn, at least 7 inches off the floor to jog in place. Maintain 550 steps per session. Remember to do an Integration Breath before next exercise. Monitor heart rate.

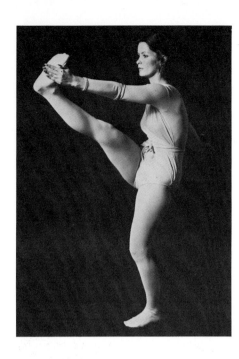

Front Roundhouse Kick

Strengthens and stretches leg muscles. Develops balance and coordination. Helps grounding. From Kung Fu.

1　Stand, feet shoulder width and parallel.
2　Kick right leg in a counterclockwise arc until leg hits left hand, extended from shoulder.
3　Repeat same procedure with left leg, this time in a clockwise arc.

Start with ten for each leg; add five per week until you reach twenty-five. The kicking leg is slightly bent, instep hitting opposite hand.

Skate

Aids balance, increases strength in legs and lower back. From yoga.

1　Standing, lift right leg into horizontal position behind you as you arch the back, lifting arms to the side for balance—fingers upward, palms facing away from you.
2　Reverse to left leg.

Balance for four deep breaths; add two breaths each week until you reach ten.

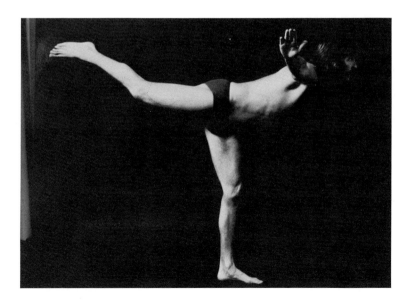

Shoulder Stand to Plough

Stimulates thyroid and parathyroid glands. Increases circulation to spinal region, stretches muscles in back of legs, soothing to nerves. This exercise should be done carefully and with caution. From yoga.

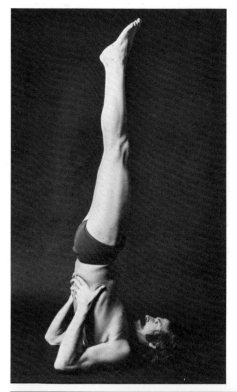

1 Go into shoulder stand (see page 57), and slowly lower both legs until toes touch the floor in back of you.
2 Slowly move arms back past head until hand touches toes (for additional stretching of spine). This is the Plough Pose. Do four deep breaths.
3 Move hands back into position, holding small of back, then return to the shoulder stand, raising legs toward sky.
4 One breath in shoulder stand before arching back into the ''Bridge to Wheel'' exercise, next in this Cycle.

Start with four deep breaths in Plough; add two each week until you reach ten.

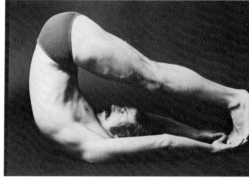

Bridge to Wheel

All benefits of back bending. Stretches spine, legs, hips, shoulders, and arms; strengthens arms. This exercise should be done carefully and with caution. From yoga.

1   After shoulder stand go into bridge pose for one deep breath. From a secure bridge pose, place palms on floor in back of shoulders, fingers facing toward body.
2   Inhale while raising pelvis. Retain 5 seconds.
3   Exhale slowly, lowering entire body. Do once.

Raise body as high as possible. Work on bringing hands closer to feet.

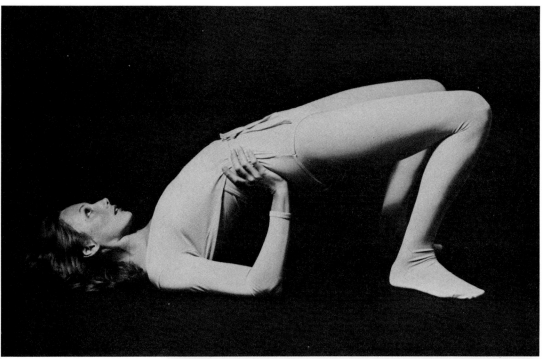

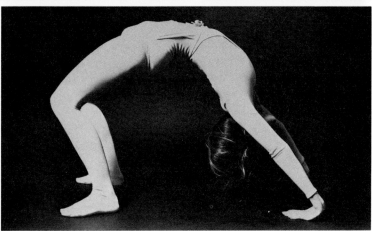

Contraction/Relaxation

Restores vitality. Do this one in the Corpse Pose.

1 Bring awareness to toes in your right foot, wiggle them and stretch them. Spread toes apart. Relax.

2 Come up to ankle; rotate ankle, creating pressure.

3 Flex calf muscles. Relax.

4 Bring awareness to thigh. Tighten it, tighten it more. Lift straightened leg off floor 2 inches, tighten, drop. Relax.

5 Roll your right leg. Become aware of toes. Repeat technique for left leg.

6 From left thigh, take awareness to right hand. Rotate thumb and fingers, open and close palm. Stretch fingers and palm. Center of palm will rise slightly. Hold for one breath. Make a fist and rotate from wrist; create pressure for one breath. Straighten arm off floor 2 inches. Tighten fist, forearm, and upper arm as tight as you can for one breath and drop. Roll.

7 Repeat with left hand and arm.

8 Contract muscles in rectum. If done correctly, your buttocks will rise from the ground. Tighten for one breath. Exhale and relax.

9 Breathe long and deep into belly. Holding breath for 3 counts, push out belly. Exhale rapidly through mouth.

10 After 10 seconds of normal breathing, expand chest. Push out from inside holding three counts, exhale rapidly through mouth.

11 Try to make shoulders meet over chest, holding for one breath; exhale and drop shoulders.

12 Move the muscles in your face, make ugly faces, phony smiles to break down the tension. Imagine a paintbrush sticking out of your chin. Paint circles and figure eights on the ceiling and walls. Bring the energy into a small ball in the center of your face trying to mash your lips against your nose. Inhale, exhale while releasing contractions in face.

13 Inhale long and deep into belly. Do not contract muscles. Imagine a white vibrational wave coming in through your toes and going out the top of your head. As you imagine this wave be aware of the different parts of your body it passes on its journey up and out the top of your head.

Contract and tense muscles as tight as you can, then release contraction and "let go" to achieve a more relaxed state. Start from your toes and think of each part of the body until you reach your head.

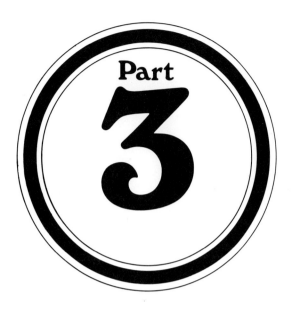

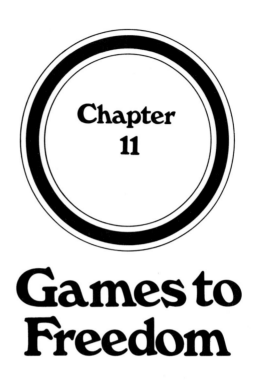

Chapter 11

Games to Freedom

We know that it is important for us to move our bodymind in different ways. We must frequently sustain movement to maintain health. Good feelings and satisfaction come from the ability to move the bodymind well. Yet it seems that there are barriers preventing us from developing this ability. They are constructed from the fear of discovery, from our own seemingly overwhelming anxieties. We must push out. If we can find and break through those barriers, relying on our own inner strength, we can ultimately become free. This applies to sports, games, and other types of body movement. Games to freedom can help.

Games to freedom are physical activities that give you a greater insight into, understanding of, and pleasure in your bodymind, augmenting the E/W program. These games are more like play than exercises, and they can help reestablish contact between you and your environment (air, earth, water, and people). Games to freedom broadens your perspective toward sports and games, making participation a richer and more rewarding experience and developing a more positive attitude toward your bodymind. Games to freedom are for having fun while integrating the inner and outer man.

As we have said, one aim of games to freedom is to change your attitude toward yourself and the way you move your body—with the result of dropping inner impediments to free expression. If you have been turned off to body movement at an early age, that doesn't mean you can't change now and still have a wonderful life of sports and games ahead of you. It may mean, in some cases, that it will take you longer to learn a particular skill. But the first obstacle is your own indifference or dislike for sports.

Sports have a tremendous influence in teaching us values of our culture and life, particularly in our early years. But conventional sports and physical education programs often serve only to reinforce a winner/loser attitude about sports. Emphasis is placed on reaching the finish line first or getting the most points. This one-dimension goal becomes an obstacle to experience, and the negative peer pressure can discourage many of us at an early age. It also stops many weekend, amateur and even professional athletes from experiencing peak bodymind-expanding performances.

We accept our competitive orientation so readily that we lose sight of some vital questions: Is the will to win only applicable in a man-against-man contest, or does it pertain as well when the only competitor is one's self? Is elapsed time the only criterion of success in a race, or is the real success the joy of the activity? Does the concentration on being first stop the understanding and the feeling of the experience between the start and finish line? Can creativity be learned through sports, or do the current rules stop any creative expansion? You can answer these questions yourself from your own experiences, or you will be able to when you understand games to freedom—games we play, not watch.

Not all sports need opponents in order to play. And not all competition needs a winner or loser. Competition can be regarded as cooperation. You need the other team or person to make the dynamics of the sport. So, in a sense, you are sharing this competitive arena in order to find out something or get something. The greatest rewards, whether in winning or losing, are coordination, balance, strength, stamina, and agility, on the one hand, and cooperation, courtesy, sportsmanship, self-reliance, emotional maturity, responsibility, and individuality, on the other.

Games to freedom helps us integrate ourselves through expanding and enriching our understanding of sports. The movements free our minds from rote thoughts and become, therefore, a kind of moving meditation.

Recent studies on the two hemispheres of the brain can shed some light on the nature of movement games to freedom. The left hemisphere is involved with verbal-analytic, logical, sequential, and rational thought. The right hemisphere is involved with spatial perception, artistic talent, crafts, body movement, and intuition. According to Dr. Roger Sperry, a psychobiologist at Cal Tech., "excellence in one tends to interfere with top level performance in the other." Dr. Robert Ornstein, a research scientist at San Francisco's Langley-Porter Institute, helps verify this point: "We've found that right-handed people, when they're, say, writing, turn on the left hemisphere—the verbal and linear side—and turn off the right hemisphere—the spatial and intuitive side—so that the two hemispheres do not interfere with each other." According to this theory, when doing certain exercises (like swimming), however, you turn on the (right) spatial-intuitive hemisphere.

Using the right side of the brain allows you to begin to perceive that the essence of the universe is within you—that intuition solves problems that are beyond the reach of your reasoning power. The opposite is true for some left-handers. The information that comes through will help you to lead a healthy life.

Ornstein adds, "The nervous system is specialized to deal with changes in the outside world and not so much with constancies, so, when you keep stimulating it in just one way, it begins to shut off its normal mode of processing. This is when we experience an altered state of consciousness."

It's not necessary to turn sports and games into a mystical experience, but we should understand that there is more to them than is taught today. We do get exhilarated while playing. We can learn about ourselves and life from the type of sports we play and how we play them—our attitude toward life. We can see, balance, and channel our aggression into sports.

The most important point is to get out and play sports—either individual or team sports. Your body type will dictate to a certain extent what sports to play, but, whatever you do, start now. Play several sports—the more moves your body learns the better it will respond on the playing field and in life. Then trust your bodymind—after it is open and free, it will always make the best choice.

The following are some games to freedom to use as a start— some new, many old, but here for the picking.

Paddle Ball

The versatility of paddle ball makes it a game that is becoming more popular. It can be played indoors and out, with rules on a regulation court or on grass or the beach without rules. Paddle ball without rules is a game that differs from most sports and games.

Most sports are played until a point is scored; then the playing is temporarily stopped, as in tennis and handball. The object is to keep the ball away from the opponent(s) in order to win the point.

In ruleless paddle ball, the golden rule is cooperation—hitting the ball back to the other player so you can continue playing. It takes just as much accuracy to hit the ball back to the other player as it does to place it out of reach of an opponent. Actually, it takes more endurance to play cooperative paddle ball because rallies last longer.

Ruleless or cooperative paddle ball is a nice way to communicate and make friends at the park or beach. It's easy to learn and fun to play. The intensity and speed are regulated by the ability of both players. The game can be played with a ball anywhere in size from a squash ball to tennis ball. Paddles range in size from Ping Pong to a regulation-size paddle. Drilling holes in the paddles helps increase the speed of the swing. Remember to exhale each time you hit the ball. (For that matter, you should also exhale when you hit or throw any ball.)

Inhale when you catch it. Paddle ball develops eye/hand coordination and concentration. Changing hands with the paddle gives the other side of the body more development and balance. Playing while running develops heart, lungs and endurance.

Frisbee

Frisbee is a way of communicating, making friends, and moving your body, sometimes in new and different ways.

The short rim of the underside of this plastic dish allows the thrower a number of different grasps in order to send the Frisbee into different flight patterns and angles. Frisbee is versatile; a game of Frisbee may demand that you leap, twirl, run, whirl, twist, and sprint while catching or throwing the flying disk. The game can incorporate a number of fitness elements—flexibility, eye/hand coordination, eye/foot coordination, speed, agility, and cardiovascular endurance.

Once you become practiced enough, you will learn to throw the Frisbee into the air at an angle which will allow it to return to you, as a boomerang would. At that proficiency, you can play any time, almost anywhere, so you don't have to wait until you find throwing partners.

A California psychiatrist, Dr. Stancil Johnson, said, "You can wind up and hurl one as hard as you want with very little chance of even stinging anyone's hand. It's great for getting rid of aggressive tendencies. It's play with a difference, and it isn't full of rules."

Nude Dance

In the privacy of your own home, apartment, or room, play your favorite music. It can be classical, rock, jazz, country—whatever suits your taste. Start to feel the music, the tempo, beat, rhythm. Slowly at your own speed start to move with the music your own way. At first you may fall into a pattern of a popular dance movement you know. That's okay for now, just so you are moving. When you feel fairly comfortable about your dance movement, begin to undress yourself slowly, one article of clothing at a time. You might even try to keep into the beat of the music while you're peeling off the clothes, but do not interrupt the rhythm of your breathing.

All sorts of funny notions are apt to flash through your mind: "This is silly"; "I can't do it"; "All my clothes? What if someone is watching?"; "This is terrific"; "I'm free—everyone should practice this!"; "I feel sexy." Try to control your mind and to imagine that you are shedding hangups that stop you from moving a certain way as you shed each article of clothing. Feel your body as you move; watch it in the mirror. Check out how your body, particularly your pelvis, is moving.

Try to move in new movements that you are unaccustomed to doing. Try movements you see other people do and you think you can't because you never really give yourself the chance. Do movements that feel uncoordinated and unsightly. You'll be surprised how these movements can develop into smooth flowing graceful actions if you work with them in a fun, positive way and don't put them aside forever as impossible.

The idea is not to make a nudist out of you, but to give you the opportunity to feel, see, touch, and move your body in new ways under circumstances not normal in your everyday life. Try to overcome your embarrassment. It is another way to start integrating outer and inner, looking into yourself.

Robot

You can play robot anywhere indoors and out, alone or in a crowd. All you need is yourself—and a certain degree of tension in the right places in your body.

You will create your own robot, but here are some suggestions to get started: walk stiff-legged; don't bend your knees unless your robot is sitting down. Even then, his legs can be straight. When turning to right or left, don't turn from your waist; turn your waist and shoulders together in one motion, along with your feet, showing how inflexible your robot really is. Every move is clumsy and jerky. The head turns in short quick turns, eyes looking straight ahead. Your entire body has a degree of rigidity to it.

Many people don't have to go too far in their bodies to realize the mechanical man. He responds the exact same way to the same stimuli. He is programmed into a pattern, the same tape is played over and over in his head. After you find your mechanical man, humanize him.

Blowing Bubbles

If you have had a fearful experience which has made you afraid of water, that fear can be alleviated. The more secure you are in the water, the easier you will learn to swim. If you already know how to swim, but you are that one scared swimmer who swims as fast as you can across the pool fighting the water the entire way across, thinking you will sink if you don't stroke quickly—this exercise can help you.

Fill up your wash basin with water a few inches from the top. Bend from the waist putting your face underwater. Rotate your head to the right so your mouth barely clears the water and inhale a deep quick breath. Turn your head back into the water and slowly blow the exhalation into the water, causing bubbles. Rotate your head to the left, mouth just above the water, inhaling quickly. Turn face back into the water slowly, exhaling and creating bubbles.

You should inhale quickly, because when swimming the crawl stroke, in which this breathing technique is used, you haven't much time to get the breath. You have all the time you need, but you must be quick. When you breathe out underwater, there is no need to be afraid of swallowing water—you are blowing *out*. The only chance for water to rush in is when you inhale underwater, and of course you can't do that unless you're a fish. You're learning that you can open your mouth underwater as long as you don't inhale. You are also learning bilateral breathing (that's breathing on both sides). This breathing technique in itself helps you balance when swimming the crawl.

Climb a Tree

Unless you live on an island where coconuts grow or you're a professional tree pruner or lumberjack, tree climbing stopped somewhere in your childhood years. Our society tells us we should outgrow many things that would be healthy to continue. Tree climbing develops strength in arms, shoulders, and hands.

We marvel at natives running up tall coconut palms when it's only a matter of technique, practiced to a skill. And let's eliminate any negative thoughts of falling out of the tree right now; you will not fall if you pay attention and concentrate on what you are doing at present: climbing a tree.

First you have to find a tree that you can climb. That means the tree must be large and sturdy enough to support your weight. It's important that its limbs be strong enough, and you must remember not to get too far out on the limb.

When you find the right tree, make sure no one owns it; if someone does, ask permission to climb it. It's funny to think someone could own a tree. Trees are for all of us to see and enjoy; but when a tree is used to climb it's better to ask.

Beware of the strength of the tree's limbs as well as your own strength. The danger comes when you are out of balance—either your limbs are not strong enough for the tree, or the tree's limbs are not strong enough for you. Be aware of height.

You will use many sets of muscles to climb—arms, hands, legs, inner thighs, feet—and become aware of the coordination between them.

Jump and Spin

This game is more like an exercise. It helps develop strength and bounce in legs, along with coordination and balance.

Feet should be shoulder width apart, knees slightly bent. Face a window, wall, tree, barn, or the sea, but whatever it is, think of it as one side of a square. Jump one quarter turn to the right, landing in the same position you started the jump, feet parallel, shoulder width apart. Practice the quarter turn jump once to the right four times and once to the left four times.

Next jump and turn 180° to the right. This is an about-face to the wall or object directly behind you. Repeat a few times to the right and then the left. You may have to use your arms to help spin you around.

Next try a three-quarter jump and spin. Here the arms come more into play. Try to land with your feet shoulder width and parallel. When you master the three-quarter jump and spin, progress to the full turn, landing where you started. Your arms, hips, shoulders, and legs all work together to spin to 360°. You may find it is easier to maintain your balance on the right or left side. Work on both sides. You can always try $1^{1}/_{4}$ and $1^{1}/_{2}$ turns when you perfect the 360°.

Two variations of the jump and spin are to start from a semisquat position and from a kneeling position.

Be an Animal

This is one of those games that work on several levels of awareness. Your imagination must work so that you can pick your first animal. Then your imagination tells you how to move in your animal's body. Sit like your animal—walk, run, trot, or lope as it does. Smell, touch, and eat as it does. An apple might be a food your animal would eat. Try drinking water the way it would.

This is a game you can play at a people-gathering. See how your animal relates to the other animals.

Pantomime Sport and Overload Training

Imagination comes into play with pantomime sport. You pretend you are in actual play in whatever sport you pick. For example, in tennis you would take your racket in hand and play an imaginary game in your backyard. Plant your feet in the same way you would for a brilliant backhand and swing to hit the imaginary ball. For basketball, dribble around an imaginary defense. Pass the ball against a wall—and then be the receiver catching the pass. Exhale on the pass, inhale on the catch.

Skills are learned through repetition. The more you do the movement the better you learn it, which leads to a better performance. Of course, there is a difference when you actually play the game; the timing will be different, and so will the pressure and excitement.

Overload training is similar to pantomime except you increase resistance to the movement by adding weight. Swinging a weighted golf club, tennis racket, or baseball bat is an example of overload training.

Tying rubber tubing around your ankles and using a small inflatable tube to keep legs afloat strengthens arms for the swimming crawl. It has been documented that, although strength and endurance are improved by overload, timing is thrown off, so bear in mind that adjustments must be made.

Walk

Walking needs no explanation, but most of us in America don't do enough of it. Long walks help develop heart and lungs. What's a long walk? That's up to you, but anything over a half hour at a steady stride gets your heart beating to cause a conditioning effect. Walking to meet a friend at the crossroads makes the action seem easier and seems to delay fatigue. Watch your breath while walking in order to develop control of the breath. It is said that, "when one controls breath, one controls life."

A simple walking, breathing exercise: count each step as you inhale to five. For the next five steps retain the breath, and the following five steps exhale. Continue as long as comfortable. After you do it a few times, you will learn how to control and regulate your breath to the steps. Increase the counts from five to whatever is comfortable. Remember to keep your feet straight and parallel, and to keep "swivel hips," loose and swinging.

Balance Walk

The balance beam is a gymnastic event in the Olympics for women. It takes a tremendous amount of coordination and balance to do the tricks these women perform. We can improve and develop our balance by walking lines on the sidewalk, walking on a fallen tree in the country, or walking the edge of a curb on a city street.

Walk backward slowly. Try to hit on your toes and the ball of your foot, touching the line with each step. Try it sideways. Make up variations. You will think of them when you start playing the game.

Blind Walk

Another way of understanding your body and how it feels to move in a different way is to walk wearing a blindfold. You might first try this in your own personal environment: apartment, home, backyard. Walk slowly using a stick, cane, or broom handle as a guide. Listen to your breathing, and breathe into your belly.

Walk/Climb a Mountain

Take a walk/climb up a mountain. Start with a mountain that's right for you. Don't look for a mountain too high or difficult. You may want to start with a hill. It doesn't matter as long as you have an experience—you and the mountain. You don't need any equipment, just a good pair of walking/climbing boots and the idea that you would like to experience this type of sport.

Your attention and awareness of magnificent views and environment, combined with increased heartbeat and oxygen intake, will create an exciting and exhilarating experience.

Run/Jog

Running/jogging is one of the best games you can play, if you have the right attitude. There is a great deal of information around today about how effective running/jogging is on cardiovascular and respiratory systems. People have gotten the message—tracks are becoming crowded—to keep heart, lungs, and skeletal muscles in good shape. However, many of these runners dislike the thought of spending the time running a boring treadmill or track, but, since they know there are benefits, they think they must follow the procedure—and they are right in part.

Let's change the boring aspects. Running is a way to discovery—inside and out. If you have discovered it is boring to run on a treadmill or track, change your running environment. Besides the element of poor weather, one of the reasons you would run a treadmill or track is because "there isn't any place to run." If you look again through eyes that have a slightly different perspective, you will probably discover an interesting, if not a different, running environment. Practically every city has a park or a lake to run around, or a residential area without many cars or buses. There is one nice thing about running outdoors in the park, country forest, or beach: the running part of you is taking the rest of you—your senses of sight, smell, touch, and hearing—on a journey of discovery. You pick the place. You may feel a bit silly in public the first few times out, but you'll get over it. Most people who say anything say something positive: "Keep going" or "I wish I were you." Smile at the occasional heckler.

If you want to run a set course every time, pick a spot where you enjoy the scenery or the spot where you feel most comfortable. It is your run—have fun with it. Let the fun of the run energize you through the setting you've chosen.

For the new runners—and there is a runner in all of us, or we would not have read this—start slowly. Run a distance or a length of time that is comfortable. Your first run could be one minute or ten minutes—it depends on you. If you aren't running to break a record or place first, you're running to enjoy it. While enjoying it, you still get the benefits of increasing heart and lung efficiency. If you need a time or distance goal, it is said someone is in good shape if he can run 1½ miles in 12 minutes. If you want to avoid a measured track, you can measure your own. Do so by driving the distance and reading the car's speedometer, or hook up a pedometer and walk the distance. To get some feedback on your progress, keep a check on your running time periodically.

"Long slow distance" is a wonderful way to start and continue a running/jogging program. You simply increase the time and distance, slowly and progressively. That is not to say you measure the distance. When do you increase? You'll know as your body builds stamina; could be a week or month.

You can even use the old Scout's pace method at first. For example, run 100 steps and walk 100 for five minutes. The next week you run 200 steps and walk 100 for five minutes. Eventually you eliminate the walk. However, when you first start, remember to breathe fully. Try breathing in through the nose and out through the mouth.

Running on a beach can have its dull and negative moments. By negative moments I mean thoughts that negate what you are doing: "I wish I was finished"; "Maybe I'll stop and rest"; "I'll walk back." We all see them pop into our bodymind now and again. There is a game that stops the "monkey chatter," as Zen would call it.

The game is "run the waterline." You have to be near a sea or ocean to play. Since waves do not break at the same time, the waterline is never straight. Like life, it's constantly changing. The game is to keep your feet or ankles dry while running inches away from the water. As the water recedes you can jog or lope down with the water, but when the next wave breaks, you must sprint to keep dry, still staying inches from the water. When playing the game it is difficult to think about being someplace else.

When you run the waterline, you may feel like a ball carrier eluding tacklers. Here you can vary running sideways, backward, discovering new ways of moving your body. In feudal Japan, the *ninja* was a master of deception. These highly trained espionage agents developed a dozen different walking and running steps. Tracks left by side walking and running did not reveal which way the *ninja* was traveling. Side running was also used to escape through narrow passages and bamboo groves. Try this method.

The Tarahumara Indians of the Sierra Madre, Mexico, are well known for their tremendous endurance and stamina. The runners (practically everyone is a runner) kick a carved wooden ball the size of a softball while they run. They run wherever they go, kicking the ball.

My friend Benny, a Taos Pueblo Indian and a distance runner, taught me to run like a rabbit—jumping, leaping from side to side. It's especially helpful when running in the country over ruts and gulleys, while constantly aware of what your next step will be.

If you find an uninhabited area to take a run, try letting out a scream as you run. Raising your hands toward the sky, open your throat and let out the scream from the pit of your stomach.

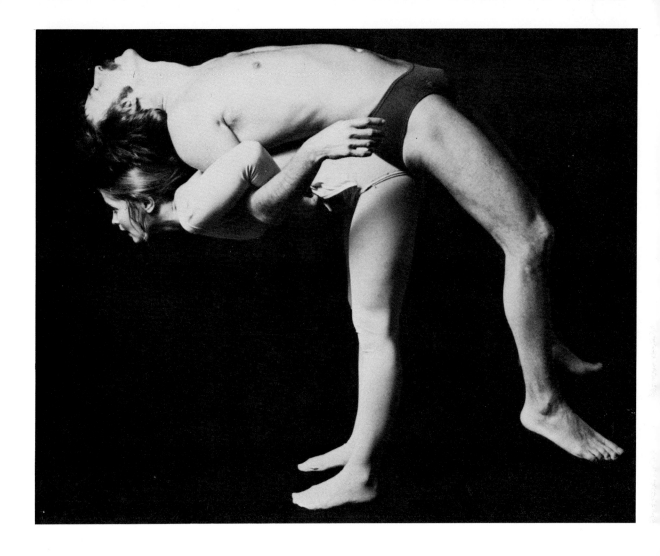

Back Relaxer

Relaxes neck and back muscles. An exercise for two.

1 Stand back to back with your partner, interlocking arms at elbows.
2 Person A bends forward at waist while Person B relaxes, leaning backward, breathing deeply, and resting on the back of Person A.
3 Reverse positions.

Hold for as long as is comfortable for both persons (around 30 seconds). Do twice.

Forward bending should be done slowly. The person on top will experience a feeling of "letting go." Person in bottom position bounces lightly, twice. It is helpful for both persons to be approximately the same height.

Sitting Seesaw

Stretches and strengthens muscles in legs, inner thighs, and small of back. An exercise for two.

1   Sitting opposite each other, both partners spread their legs as wide as possible. The bottoms of each partner's feet should touch.
2   Holding hands, arms out, parallel to floor. Person A slowly leans back, pulling Person B forward. Hold for one breath.
3   Reverse, Person B slowly leaning back, pulling Person A forward. Hold for one breath and continue.

Start with five pulls, adding three a week until you reach fifteen.

Partners may have different stretching capacities. Be aware of this so you aren't pulled—and don't pull your partner—past the stretching limit too quickly.

Remember to move slowly.

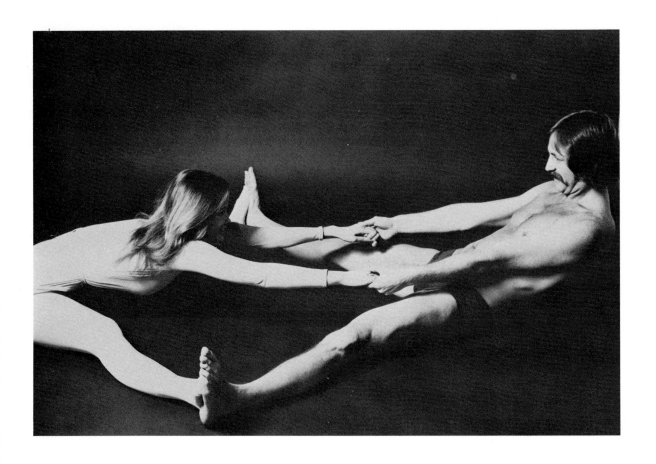

Drownproofing

Drownproofing is a method of staying afloat easily for long periods of time. This method, created by Fred Lanoue, uses principles of breath control and energy conservation. It is a good idea to learn drownproofing in case you should ever need it, as well as for the experience. Even poor swimmers who learn the technique can stay afloat for hours. Just be cautious and careful while you learn this technique. The best place is a pool with a lifeguard on duty.

Here is Lanoue's technique:

1 With the lungs full of air, float face down, arms and legs dangling downward, with the back of the neck on the surface.

2 Get ready for a slow, easy, downward push, using arms, legs or both. Bring arms up slowly, hands crisscrossed in front of mouth and nose, palms facing outward.

3 Exhale through the nose while (*not* before and *not* after) raising the head just high enough to get the chin out of the water. Keep shoulders under water.

4 The instant the head is vertical, bring your arms downward and outward (across your body), making the downward thrust which supports the body during the inhalation through the mouth.

5 As soon as the lungs are full, drop the face down to the horizontal, bring the arms up slowly, each hand crisscrossed across nose and face, palms outward, and immediately give another long, slow thrust backward and downward.

6 Relax with head, arms, and legs dangling, holding all air for 4 or 5 seconds while slowly floating forward and upward.

Swimming at the Ocean

Swimming at a beach where there is strong undertow can be treacherous. The undertow can sometimes take your legs out from under you. There are times when even strong swimmers are quickly pulled away from the shoreline by the riptide.

It works like this: the surf constantly breaks against the shore in waves. Some of this volume of water returns to the ocean underneath the breaking waves; the rest of the water returns in a trough or channel called a riptide.

If caught in a riptide, the first reaction—especially in the state of panic—is to sprint straight for the beach. If you find you have not got the strength and stamina, swim parallel to the beach in order to get out of the riptide. Once past the riptide, swim toward the beach, and the chances are you'll be helped into shore by the next wave.

Chapter 12

Exercises for Office and School

A healthy person needs less energy to work, study, or play than an unfit person. The healthier you are the more energy you'll have to do everyday activities without fatigue. Change your sedentary work or study place into a space that can be fun—and at the same time benefit you by the increased capacity to get more work done easier.

You can learn and develop an entire series of exercises done throughout the day—rising, dressing, commuting, working/studying—to supplement your E/W program. Doing these exercises while at work is almost like being paid to keep fit, and everyone benefits. There are always a few moments at work or school that can be filled with exercise; it's fun and easy, and there's no lack of time.

Some of these exercises are merely everyday activities done in such a way that the activity becomes a beneficial exercise, for example, tightening and relaxing muscles in abdomen and buttocks at a stop light (while commuting) or at the sound of a horn and/or telephone, holding a telephone receiver with isometric pressure, using your desk and chair as exercise apparatus.

You will find there are many ways to exercise within the limitations of your daily activities. After using the exercises shown here you will develop more exercises adapted for your specific needs in your place of work or study.

We already know that it is best to do the E/W program at the same time and place each day. Your wake-up, commute, and office/school exercises work are the same. Start with a few exercises and add new ones as the old become positive habits.

Here's how it works:

Get-Up Exercises
Do any or all of these. In bed or lying on the floor, raise head, shoulders, and legs 6 inches off the floor or bed. Arms straight, palms down, point fingers toward toes, which should be held straight.

Do twenty Breaths of Fire.

Roll in a ball ten times (see page 107).

While Brushing Teeth, Shaving, or Brushing Hair
Pull in abdominal muscles (navel toward spinal column). Tighten buttocks. Hold each for count of three breaths.

While getting dressed, move the face muscles in ways they don't ordinarily move. Make ugly faces and phony smiles, then relax.

While Traveling

Try to walk or bicycle to work/school. If you commute by car, bus, subway, or train, pull in abdominal muscles at stop light or scheduled stops. Get off mode of transportation far enough from work/school site to walk a good distance.

Pull in abdominal muscles and/or tighten buttocks when you hear a car horn.

Each week, increase the distance you walk, but do not increase the amount of time needed to complete walk.

Get off elevator several floors below your floor and walk the rest of the way.

Start skipping every other stair and increase to every third stair.

You will now be more alert at your office or school. And you can do the same exercises on the way home. At first you can write exercises on little slips of paper as reminders. Put them in or on the places where you do the particular exercise. Start with a specific area that needs firming or stretching, then add to the list.

Exercises to Do at Work or School

When doing isometric exercises—pushing against an immovable object—slowly ease into the holding position, hold for three long, deep breaths, then ease off. Don't hold your breath—hold your muscles. Be in control.

Sitting at your desk or standing, clasp hands in back of your head. Try to push your head backward as you resist with your hands. Do this in three positions:

1 Head down, eyes looking at floor.
2 Eyes straight.
3 Eyes looking at ceiling.

Reverse the pressure with hands on forehead and do same three positions. Remember to ease into a hold for three breaths.

The following exercises for office and school were chosen to aid the parts of your body listed in the margin.

Place hand on side of head, try to push your ear to shoulder. Resist with pressure from hand. Do both sides. Sitting at desk or standing, slowly roll your head. This exercise reduces headaches and neck tension.

For Neck

For Shoulders	Sitting at your desk, place the back of hand under the front lip of your desk (arms straight). Pushing up, try and lift up desk. Hold for three breaths; repeat twice. Reverse and try to lift desk with your palms up.
For Arms, Shoulders, and Chest	Sitting in your chair, do a modified shoulder bounce (see page 48), while grasping the seat of the chair. Lift shoulders and hold for three breaths. Do twice.
	Use your desk to do pushups, both forward and backward. You already know the forward pushup. Hold onto the front of the desk, feet back 3 or 4 feet, and begin. In the backward pushup, you turn around, with your back facing the desk, walk forward about 3 feet from desk. Holding onto desk, slowly push off, arching back. Hold for three breaths and return. Do three times. Grasp the arms or the seat of your chair and push straight up and off chair. Hold and return. Do three. A variation of this is to straighten legs out in front, then lift off chair (also good for abdominals).
	Standing in front of filing cabinet, one hand on each side, try to push hands together. Hold three breaths. After a telephone conversation, place both hands on receiver; try to pull it apart. Hold. The reverse of this is to push the receiver together. Do each three times.
For Upper Arms	Sit close enough to your desk to flex elbows into an L shape, with palms under desk. Try to lift desk. Hold three breaths. Do three times.
For Back	Standing, bend at waist, place hands behind knees, fingers facing each other. Pull in abdominal muscles and try to straighten your back. Resist with your hands, hold. Do twice.
	Stand next to desk. Lean over desk; hold onto it with hands. Raise one leg (keep straight) slowly as high as possible. Hold three breaths. Return to floor. Repeat with other leg. (A variation can be done with one leg bent.)
For Back and Waist	Sitting at desk, feet together, touch toes with hands, placing head on knees. Hold for three breaths.

Sitting at desk, cross one leg over the other at ankle. Hands hold onto seat, or arms of chair. Lift one leg with the other. Switch legs. Lift each leg five times.

For Abdominals, Hips, Thighs, and Buttocks

When the telephone or class bell rings, pull in abdominals and/or buttocks muscles. Hold for five breaths; if you are talking on the phone, hold for a comparable time. (You *can* hold and talk at the same time.)

Sitting at desk, feet together, twist arms and shoulders to left, knees and legs to the right; feel twist at waist. Do three times on each side.

Sitting at desk, feet together, holding chair seat or arms of chair, lift one knee at a time as high as possible. Three times each leg.

Sitting at desk, feet together, holding seat or arms of chair, straighten, legs slowly, raising legs as high as possible, then slowly return feet to floor. Do three times.

Sitting at desk, legs straight out, alternate legs, bringing knee to chest. Three times each.

Sitting at desk, legs straight out, do scissors ten times.

Sitting at desk, legs straight out, do the flutter kick ten times.

Sitting at desk, feet on floor, knees at either side of desk well, push out and hold three breaths. For similar results on thighs, without using a desk, place feet 18 inches apart, place right hand on outside of right knee, left hand on outside of left knee, try to push knees apart, resisting with hand.

Sitting at desk, knees on either side of a sturdy wastebasket, push in. Or place feet 18 inches apart, cross your arms (i.e., place right hand on inside of left knee and left hand on inside of right knee). Try to squeeze knees together, resisting with hands.

Standing (alone, waiting in line, etc.), slowly rise on your toes as high as possible; hold; return to floor. Do three times.

For Legs and Feet

Use the stairs more each day.

Feel the bottom of your feet making contact with the floor when you rise from your chair.

Studying at home, barefoot, pick up marbles or pencil with toes.

Sitting at desk, legs straight, toes pointed, make a circle with foot, clockwise, then counterclockwise, creating pressure at ankle.

The following exercises are familiar ones, taken from the cycles listed at the left:

Sitting at a Desk

Remember to keep back straight while sitting.

From Cycle	Exercise
	Breath of Fire
	Head/Neck Roll
I	Petoral Press
	Contraction/Relaxation (modified for sitting)
	Cooling Breath
	Book Lift (modified for sitting)
II	Energy Ball
	Contraction/Relaxation (Short Form) (modified for sitting)
	Complete Breath
III	Neck Stretch
	Pushup Sleeve
	Lion
	Cleansing Breath
	Camel Neck Roll
IV	Wrist Circles
	Abdominal Pump (modified)
	Eye Exercise
	Alternate Breathing
V	Look Left/Turn Right
	Fingers Back

Standing

From Cycle	Exercise	From Cycle	Exercise
	Breath of Fire		Complete Breath
	Sky/Earth		Egyptian Stretch
	Head/Neck Roll		Sky/Earth Picking
	Shoulder Bounce		Apples/Touch Heels
	Pectoral Press		Neck Stretch
	Trunk Lateral Bend		Shoulder Roll
I	Slow Twist		Pushup Sleeve
	Jump Rope or	III	Ax Twist
	Run in Place		Hip Swing
	Knee to Chest		Lateral Walk
	Squat Stand		Jump Rope or
	Integration Breath		Run in Place No. 3
			Pendulum Kick
	Cooling Breath		Masai Stand
	Sky/Earth Picking Apples		Lion
	Arm Circles		
	Book Lift (modified for standing)		Cleansing Breath
	Broom Twist		Sky/Earth Picking Apples/Hip-Up
	Energy Ball		Camel Neck Roll
	Bump/Ground Rotation		Shoulder Roll/
II	Balance Sway		Waist Bend
	Jump Rope No. 2 or		Pullup
	Run in Place		Top Twist
	Hamstring Stretch	IV	Wrist Circles
	Squat Stand/		Abdominal Pump
	Buttocks Up		Push Air
	Contraction/Relaxation (Short Form) (modified for standing)		Body Swings
			Knee to Chest/
			Kick Out
			Archer
			Eye Exercise
			Bioenergetic Bend
			The Stretch
			Look Left/Turn Right
			Swimmer
		V	Pull Back Fingers
			Jump Rope (Speed)/Run in Place No. 4
			Front Roundhouse Kick
			Skate

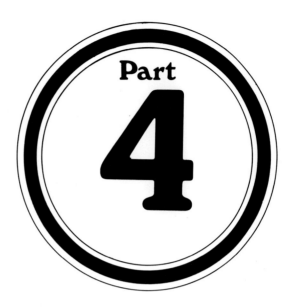

Part

4

Chapter 13

Help for Special Problems— A Ready Reference

The following list can be used as a quick reference for exercises that benefit special areas on which you wish to concentrate. Wait until you finish two or three cycles before you start working with exercises in a more demanding cycle. Your body will be better able to respond to the exercises. If an exercise is too difficult at first, drop it for the present—eventually you will be ready to learn it. If there is any question as to the effect of the exercise, consult your physician.

Abdomen

(Strengthens and firms
the upper and lower abdomen.)

From Cycle	Exercise
I	Situp No. 1
	Forward Stretch
	V Raise No. 1
	Jump Rope or Run in Place
II	Situp No. 2
	Half Locust
	Forward Stretch
	V Raise No. 2
	Jump Rope No. 2 or Run in Place No. 2
III	Situp/Knees to Chest
	Forward Stretch Groin
	V Raise No. 3
IV	Leg Swing
	Reverse Pushup
	Leg Scissors
	Forward Stretch/Foot on Thigh
	Abdominal Pump
V	Leg Circles
	Forward Stretch/ Wha Guru
	Pelvic Bounce/Arch/ Leg Raise
	Jackknife

Ankles

(Aids flexibility, strengthens, and relieves tension.)

From Cycle	Exercise
I	Rock Pose
	Slow Twist
	Jump Rope or Run in Place
	Squat Stand
II	Rock Pose/Energy Ball
	Camel Ride (Rock Pose)
	Jump Rope No. 2 or Run in Place No. 2
III	Wrists Up/Down/Rock Pose
	Lateral Walk
	Jump Rope or Run in Place No. 3
IV	Forward Stretch/Foot on Thigh
	Push Air
	Body Swings
V	Squat Lateral/Ball
	Jump Rope (Speed) or Run in Place No. 4

Arms

(Develops, strengthens, and firms.)

From Cycle	Exercise
I	Salute to the Sun
	Pushup No. 1
II	Arm Circles
	Pushup No. 2
	Energy Ball
III	Pushup No. 3
	Wrists Up/Down/Rock Pose
IV	Salute to the Sun with Dip
	Pullup
	Reverse Pushup
	Wrist Circles/Rock Pose
V	The Sprinter
	Pull Back Fingers/Rock Pose

Back

(Relieves tension;
strengthens and firms.)

From Cycle	Exercise
	Shoulder Bounce
	Situp No. 1
	Cobra
I	Camel Ride
	V Raise No. 1
	Mule Kick and Arch
	Shoulder Stand
	Situp No. 2
	Half Locust
	Camel Ride
	(Rock Pose)
II	V Raise No. 2
	Bump/Ground Rotation
	Shoulder Stand/
	Leg Bounce
	Bridge
	Egyptian Stretch
III	Bow
	V Raise No. 3
	Shoulder Roll/Waist
	Bend
	Leg Swing
	Pullup
IV	Leg Scissors
	Opposite Arm/Leg
	Raise
	Pelvic Bounce/Arch
	Up
	Archer
	Bioenergetic Bend
	The Sprinter
	Swimmer
	Squat Lateral/Ball
	Leg Circles
	Forward Stretch
	Wha Guru
V	Pelvic Bounce/Arch/
	Leg Raise
	Jackknife
	Cat and Cow
	Skate
	Shoulder Stand to Plough
	Bridge to Wheel

Balance

(Promotes equilibrium, poise,
and grace.)

From Cycle	Exercise
	Jump Rope
I	Knee to Chest
	Shoulder Stand
	V Raise No. 2
	Balance Sway
II	Jump Rope No. 2
	Shoulder Stand/
	Leg Bounce
	Bridge
	V Raise No. 3
	Lateral Walk
III	Jump Rope
	Pendulum Kick
	Masai Stand
	Head Stand
	Sky/Earth Picking
	Apples/Hip-Up
	Push Air
IV	Body Swings
	Knee to Chest/Kick-Out
	Archer
	Headstand No. 2
	Pushup/Hand Stand
	Jump Rope (Speed)
	Front Roundhouse
V	Kick
	Skate
	Shoulder Stand
	to Plough
	Bridge to Wheel

Brain

(Increases blood supply.)

From Cycle	Exercise
I	Shoulder Stand
II	Shoulder Stand/ Leg Bounce
III	Head Stand
IV	Head Stand
V	Shoulder Stand to Plough Bridge to Wheel

Breathing

(Stimulates.)

From Cycle	Exercise
I	Breath of Fire
	Jump Rope or Run in Place
	Integration Breath
II	Cooling Breath
	Jump Rope or
	Run in Place No. 2
III	Complete Breath
	Pelvic Bounce
	Hip Swing
	Jump Rope or
	Run in Place No. 3
IV	Cleansing Breath
	Abdominal Pump
	Push Air
	Body Swings
V	Alternate Breathing
	Bioenergetic Bend
	Jump Rope (Speed) or
	Run in Place No. 4

Bust and Chest

(Helps strengthen and firm.)

From Cycle	Exercise
	Pectoral Press
I	Pushup
	Run in Place
	Book Lift
II	Pushup No. 2
	Run in Place No. 2
III	Pushup Sleeve
	Pushup No. 3
IV	Pullup
V	Pushup/Hand Stand

Buttocks

(Firms buttocks muscles.)

From Cycle	Exercise
I	Cobra
II	Locust
IV	Opposite Arm/
	Leg Raise
	Archer

Calves

(Strengthens calves and
relieves leg-muscle tension.)

From Cycle	Exercise
I	Salute to the Sun Rock Pose
II	Balance Sway
III	Lateral Walk Pendulum Kick
IV	Push Air Body Swings

Circulation

(Increases circulation.)

From Cycle	Exercise
I	Breath of Fire Sky/Earth Salute to the Sun Jump Rope or Run in Place Shoulder Stand
II	Sky/Earth Picking Apples Jump Rope or Run in Place No. 2 Shoulder Stand/ Leg Bounce
III	Sky/Earth Picking Apples/Touch Heels Jump Rope or Run in Place No. 3 Head Stand
IV	Sky/Earth Picking Apples/Hip-Up Abdominal Pump Body Swings Head Stand
V	Alternate Breathing Jump Rope (Speed) or Run in Place No. 4 Shoulder Stand to Plough

Constipation

(Helps relieve constipation.)

From Cycle	Exercise
I	Forward Stretch Camel Ride
II	Forward Stretch Breath of Fire Camel Ride (Rock Pose) Squat Stand/Buttocks Up
III	Bow Forward Stretch Groin Head Stand
IV	Opposite Arm/ Leg Raise Forward Stretch/Foot on Thigh Abdominal Pump Head Stand
V	Squat Lateral/Ball

Coordination

(Aids coordination.)

From Cycle	Exercise
I	Slow Twist Jump Rope
II	Balance Sway Jump Rope
III	Situp/Knees to Chest Coordination Jump Rope
IV	Sky/Earth Picking Apples/Hip-Up Opposite Arm/ Leg Raise
V	Look Left/Turn Right Coordination Jump Rope (Speed) Front Roundhouse Kick

Endurance

(Increases endurance and stamina.)

From Cycle	Exercise
I	Jump Rope or Run in Place
II	Jump Rope or Run in Place No. 2
III	Jump Rope or Run in Place No. 3
IV	Body Swings
V	Jump Rope (Speed) or Run in Place No. 4

Energy

(Helps to increase vitality.)

From Cycle	Exercise
I	Breath of Fire Salute to the Sun Jump Rope or Run in Place Squat Stand Shoulder Stand Contraction/Relaxation Corpse Pose Shake
II	Camel Ride (Rock Pose) Jump Rope or Run in Place No. 2 Shoulder Stand/ Leg Bounce
III	Complete Breath Jump Rope or Run in Place No. 3 Lion
IV	Cleansing Breath Roll in Ball Pelvic Bounce/Arch Up
V	Bioenergetic Bend The Sprinter Jump Rope (Speed) or Run in Place No. 4

Eyes

(Strengthens and relieves
tension in eye muscles.)

From Cycle	Exercise
III	Lion
IV	Eye Exercise

Face

(Firms muscles, circulates
blood flow; relieves tension.)

From Cycle	Exercise
I	Shoulder Stand Contraction/Relaxation
II	Shoulder Stand/ Leg Bounce Contraction/Relaxation (Short Form)
III	Head Stand Lion
IV	Camel Neck Roll (for chin) Head Stand Eye Exercise
V	Shoulder Stand to Plough Bridge to Wheel

Feet

(Strengthens foot muscles.)

From Cycle	Exercise
I	Jump Rope or Run in Place Squat Stand
II	Jump Rope or Run in Place No. 2
III	Lateral Walk Jump Rope or Run in Place No. 3
V	Jump Rope (Speed) or Run in Place No 4.

Grounding

(Helps achieve grounding.)

From Cycle	Exercise
I	Forward Stretch Slow Twist Jump Rope or Run in Place Squat Stand
II	Forward Stretch/ Breath of Fire Bump/Ground Rotation Balance Sway Jump Rope or Run in Place No. 2 Squat Stand/Buttocks Up
III	Ax Twist Forward Stretch Groin Lateral Walk Jump Rope or Run in Place No. 3 Pendulum Kick Masai Stand
IV	Top Twist Forward Stretch/Foot on Thigh Push Air Body Swings Knee to Chest/Kick-Out Archer
V	Bioenergetic Bend The Stretch Squat Lateral Ball Forward Stretch Wha Guru Jump Rope or Run in Place No. 4 Front Roundhouse Kick Skate

Headaches

(Helps relieve headaches.)

From Cycle	Exercise
I	Breath of Fire Head/Neck Roll
III	Neck Stretch Head Stand
IV	Camel Neck Roll Head Stand Eye Exercise
V	Look Left/Turn Right

Heart

(Strengthens heart muscles.)

From Cycle	Exercise
I	Jump Rope or Run in Place
II	Jump Rope or Run in Place No. 2
III	Jump Rope or Run in Place No. 3
IV	Body Swings
V	Jump Rope or Run in Place No. 4

Hips

(Firms the hips.)

From Cycle	Exercise
I	Knee Bounce
II	Head to Feet Bounce Half Locust Balance Sway
IV	Sky/Earth Picking Apples/Hip-Up
V	Empty Saddle Bags

Legs

(Strengthens legs and relieves tension in leg muscles.)

From Cycle	Exercise
I	Sky/Earth Jump Rope or Run in Place
II	Sky/Earth Picking Apples Balance Sway Jump Rope or Run in Place No. 2 Hamstring Stretch Squat Stand/Buttocks Up
III	Sky/Earth Picking Apples/Touch Heels Ax Twist Lateral Walk Jump Rope or Run in Place No. 3 Pendulum Kick Masai Stand
IV	Sky/Earth Picking Apples/Hip-Up Top Twist Push Air Body Swings Knee to Chest Kick-Out
V	The Sprinter Squat Lateral/Ball Pelvic Bounce/Arch/ Leg Raise Jump Rope (Speed) or Run in Place No. 4 Front Roundhouse Kick Skate

Lungs

(Increases lung capacity.)

From Cycle	Exercise
I	Breath of Fire Jump Rope or Run in Place
II	Cooling Breath Jump Rope or Run in Place No. 2
III	Complete Breath Jump Rope or Run in Place No. 3
IV	Cleansing Breath Body Swing
V	Alternate Breath Jump Rope (Speed) or Run in Place No. 4

Neck

(Relieves neck tension and strengthens neck muscles.)

From Cycle	Exercise
I	Sky/Earth Head/Neck Roll
II	Sky/Earth Picking Apples Arm Swing
III	Sky/Earth Picking Apples/Touch Heels Head Stand
IV	Sky/Earth Picking Apples/Hip-Up Camel Neck Roll Head Stand
V	The Stretch

Nervous System

(Helps relieve
general nervous tension.)

From Cycle	Exercise
I	Breath of Fire Head/Neck Roll Contraction/Relaxation Corpse Pose
II	Broom Twist Contraction/Relaxation (Short Form)
III	Complete Breath
IV	Cleansing Breath
V	Alternate Breathing Forward Stretch Wha Guru

Pelvic Area

(Restores flexibility and relieves
tension in the pelvic area.)

From Cycle	Exercise
I	Knee Bounce Camel Ride Mule Kick and Arch Slow Twist Squat Stand
II	Head to Feet Bounce Camel Ride (Rock Pose) Bump/Ground Rotation Squat Stand/Buttocks Up Bridge
III	Pelvic Bounce Hip Swing Pendulum Kick
IV	Sky/Earth Picking Apples/Hip-Up Top Twist Pelvic Bounce Pelvic Rotation Push Air Knee to Chest Kick-Out
V	Bioenergetic Bend Pelvic Bounce/Arch/Leg Raise Cat and Cow Front Roundhouse Kick Bridge to Wheel

Posture

(Improves posture.)

From Cycle	Exercise
I	Sky/Earth Slow Twist
II	Sky/Earth Picking Apples Broom Twist
IV	Sky/Earth Picking Apples/Touch Heels
V	Push Air

Relaxation

(Aids relaxation
by reducing tension.)

From Cycle	Exercise
I	Salute to the Sun (done slowly) Contraction/Relaxation Integration Breath Corpse Pose Shake
II	Contraction/Relaxation (Short Form)
III	Camel Neck Roll
IV	Alternate Breathing

Scalp

(Stimulates the scalp.)

From Cycle	Exercise
I	Shoulder Stand Fish
II	Shoulder Stand/ Leg Bounce
III	Head Stand
IV	Head Stand
V	Shoulder Stand to Plough

Sex

(Relieves pelvic tension
and increases endurance.)

From Cycle	Exercise
I	Knee Bounce Camel Ride Mule Kick and Arch
II	Camel Ride (Rock Pose) Bump/Ground Rotation Bridge
III	Pelvic Bounce Hip Swing Pendulum Kick
IV	Pelvic Bounce/Arch Up Pelvic Rotation
V	Cat and Cow Bridge to Wheel

Shoulders

(Strengthens shoulder muscles and relieves tension.)

From Cycle	Exercise
I	Sky/Earth Shoulder Bounce Pushup No. 1
II	Sky/Earth Picking Apples Arm Swing Pushup No. 2 Broom Twist Energy Ball
III	Sky/Earth Picking Apples/Touch Heels Shoulder Roll Pushup No. 3
IV	Sky/Earth Picking Apples/Hip-Up Shoulder Roll-Bend Pullup Reverse Pushup Wrist Circles/ Rock Pose
V	Swimmer Pushup/Hand Stand Squat Lateral/Ball Coordination

Sleep

(Helps to relieve insomnia.)

From Cycle	Exercise
I	Salute to the Sun (done slowly) Contraction/Relaxation
II	Contraction/Relaxation (Short Form)
III	Alternate Breathing

Spine

(Increases flexibility and suppleness.)

From Cycle	Exercise
I	Sky/Earth Cobra Salute to the Sun Trunk Lateral Bend Mule Kick and Arch Slow Twist Shoulder Stand Fish
II	Head to Feet Bounce Sky/Earth Picking Apples Broom Twist Half Locust Camel Ride (Rock Pose) Hamstring Stretch Shoulder Stand/ Leg Bounce Bridge
III	Egyptian Stretch Sky/Earth Picking Apples/Touch Heels Ax Twist Bow Hip Swing
IV	Roll in Ball Sky/Earth Picking Apples/Hip-Up Salute to the Sun with Dip Leg Swing Pelvic Bounce/Arch Up Push Air
V	Bioenergetic Bend The Stretch The Sprinter Squat Lateral/Ball Forward Stretch Wha Guru Pelvic Bounce/ Arch/Leg Raise Cat and Cow Skate Shoulder Stand to Plough Bridge Wheel

Stomach

(Stimulates stomach function.)

From Cycle	Exercise
I	Forward Stretch
II	Forward Stretch/ Breath of Fire Bow
III	Forward Stretch Groin Head Stand
IV	Opposite Arm/ Leg Raise Forward Stretch/Foot to Thigh Abdominal Pump
V	Forward Stretch Wha Guru

Thighs

(Firms and strengthens.)

From Cycle	Exercise
I	Knee Bounce Knee to Chest Squat Stand
II	Head to Feet Bounce Half Locust Camel Ride (Rock Pose) Bump/Ground Rotation Balance Sway Hamstring Stretch Squat Stand/ Buttocks Up
III	Egyptian Stretch V Raise No. 3 Lateral Walk Pendulum Kick
IV	Top Twist Push Air Body Swings Archer
V	Empty Saddle Bags Squat Lateral/Ball Leg Circles Jackknife

Thyroid

(Benefits thyroid action.)

From Cycle	Exercise
I	Head/Neck Roll Shoulder Stand Fish
II	Shoulder Stand Bridge

Varicose Veins in Legs

(Helps relieve this condition.)

From Cycle	Exercise
I	Shoulder Stand
II	Shoulder Stand/ Leg Bounce
III	Head Stand
IV	Head Stand
V	Shoulder Stand to Plough

Waist

(Helps firm waist muscles.)

From Cycle	Exercise
I	Trunk Lateral Bend Situp No. 1 V Raise No. 1
II	Situp No. 2 V Raise No. 2
III	Situp/Knees to Chest V Raise No. 3
IV	Top Twist Abdominal Pump
V	Squat Lateral/Ball Leg Circles

Weight

(Will reduce weight, when combined with proper nutrition.)

From Cycle	Exercise
I	Situp No. 1 V Raise No. 1 Jump Rope or Run in Place
II	Cooling Breath Situp No. 2 V Raise No. 2 Jump Rope or Run in Place No. 2
III	Situp/Knees to Chest V Raise No. 3 Jump Rope or Run in Place No. 3
IV	Leg Scissors Body Swings
V	Squat Lateral/Ball Leg Circles Jump Rope (Speed) or Run in Place No. 4

Wrists

(Helps strengthen wrist muscles.)

From Cycle	Exercise
I	Jump Rope
II	Energy Ball Jump Rope
III	Wrists Up/Down/Rock Pose Jump Rope
IV	Wrist Circles/Rock Pose
V	Fingers Back/Rock Pose

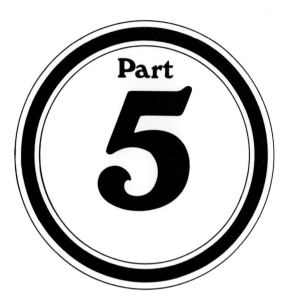

Part

5

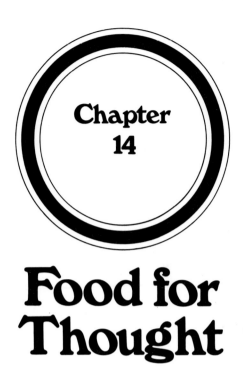

Chapter 14

Food for Thought

To begin a new and extensive exercise program you must pay attention to the quantity and quality of the food you eat. But you will find there are many conflicting ideas, theories, and diets in nutrition.

Many nutritionists are in direct disagreement. For example, some say milk is one of the major contributors to dis-ease in this country, good only for calves, kids, goats, kittens, and babies, and not for adults; they say that it causes fat and mucus, and is hard to digest, that pasteurization burns up enzymes that might have positive value. Others say that milk, specifically certified raw milk, is a good source of protein and calcium and that the yogis in India claim milk is one of the highest-level foods. All say theirs is the only way. Remember, however, that we are all unique individuals with substantially different bodies and chemical make ups, living in totally different environments—so one man's food really may be another man's poison.

This is primarily an exercise book, and I do not claim expertise in nutrition; therefore I will provide only guidelines and fundamental information about nutrition. It is a most important factor of our vitality.

One way of contributing to health is to strike a balance of right actions, thoughts, and foods. What you think, do, and eat should be in balance.

One of the first things to do is watch what you eat for a week or so. If you start the day off with coffee and donuts or use a candy bar as an afternoon pick-me-up, the sugar will give you a quick energy boost because the body uses it quickly—*then* you will crash to a lower point than that from which you started. This type of sugar causes your pancreas to release more insulin into your bloodstream, which drops your blood sugar level lower than it was before you ate the snack. This blood sugar drop accounts for the feelings of depression many sugar users experience. Instead of a quick snack, substitute protein foods—meats, fish, milk, cheese, eggs, whole grain cereals, nuts. They are broken down into a usable energy form more slowly. Energy from them builds slowly, levels to a stable high.

Look at the food while you eat. Pay attention to how the food is prepared—fried, baked, boiled, etc.—and note your eating habits. Do you dig right into a meal or pause a moment? How fast or slowly do you eat? How much do you eat? Do you eat when you are hungry or at a standard time, even if you're not? You may have to change these habits.

These are patterns of action you have learned over the years. Eating in many cases has been regarded as a source of emotional security. Your attitude toward types of food often reflects those of your parents, and perhaps its use as reward or punishment. Overindulgence and waste, we think, is a reward; it is a cultural sign of affluence and wealth, but all too often the results are punishments to the body.

Many times crash diets only work for a short time; then you may revert to the same old habits. It's wiser and more success- ful to change eating habits slowly, dropping one at a time. So if you are the type of person who needs gradual change, do it your way. Don't become a nutritional martyr—uptight about what you can or cannot eat.

Some eating suggestions:

Do not eat immediately before or after physical work or exercise. Your bodymind needs a chance to rest before eating. After eating, blood runs to the stomach and intestines to aid digestion, leaving head and limbs momentarily out of action. While doing sustained activity, take easily digested foods.

Do not eat when you are not hungry. Just because the clock says you should be hungry doesn't mean that you are. Eating by the clock is another form of overeating. Avoid stuffing yourself, so that you leave the table feeling uncomfortable or hardly able to move.

Avoid refined processed foods: white flour, white rice, milled cereals, milled and bleached breads. Foods containing chemi- cals, additives, preservatives, dyes, bleaches, conditioners, colorings, flavorings, etc., lack bulk and fiber, and they are low in nature's real food elements needed for proper cellular balance. Start to read the labels to know ingredients and eliminate as many of these artificial ones as possible.

Avoid drinking with your meals. Liquids dilute digestive en- zymes.

Avoid adding salt to already prepared foods. Salt is a mineral needed to work with potassium and helps keep calcium in solution, but there is plenty of salt in natural foods and you can replace it with powdered kelp or vegetable salt seasoning. In excess, salt is a stimulant, temporarily elevating the blood pressure and stimulating the adrenal glands. Salt overworks kidneys and interferes with the elimination of uric acids. Uric acid in the blood acts as a hindrance to circulation.

Do not eat when upset. When tense, the capillaries constrict in your digestive organs and the most nutritious foods may rot in your stomach.

Avoid coffee. Caffeine affects heart, blood pressure, liver, and kidney function if used excessively.

Avoid tobacco. We all know the story on smoking. Tobacco contains nicotine and arsenic, which are poisons.

Avoid soft drinks. If they are not full of processed sugar, they are made of chemicals. Try fruit juices.

And then there is white sugar. Overconsumption can lead to B-vitamin deficiency. It also depletes calcium in the body. It is a major cause of obesity—which is one of the major sources of heart ailments. Admittedly, it is difficult to get away from this culprit. If you have even a minor sweet tooth, refined sugar plays a major role in snack foods. Brown sugar, sometimes called "raw sugar" at the health food stores, is only white sugar dyed with molasses. If you must use sweeteners, black strap molasses and honey are better. But, for snacks, change to the natural sweets of fruits.

Foods like meat, butter, milk, and eggs in your diet are said to lead to a concentration of cholesterol in the blood. Research is beginning to lift total criticism for arteriosclerosis (hardening of the arteries) or atherosclerosis from cholesterol (which the body manufactures itself and is required for many bodily functions). Unless your serum cholesterol is high at this moment, it certainly is better to concern yourself with your whole diet rather than with reduction of cholesterol specifically.

Eat at least 50% raw food in your daily intake. Fresh raw foods, such as vegetables and fruits, are living foods and sources of concentrated vitamins, minerals, enzymes, and proteins.

Cooking and heating destroys enzymes and vitamins. Enzymes are catalysts that make the chemical changes to prepare the food for digestion and assimilation.

Chew food thoroughly. Digestion (especially of sugar and starch) begins in the mouth.

Eat whole natural foods: whole grain breads, brown rice, nuts, and soy beans (which are high in protein).

Drink fresh fruit and vegetable juices. Drink fruit juice as soon as possible after preparation, since oxygenation destroys vital enzymes.

Eat, for one day a week, only fresh fruit or vegetables. Give your system a rest and cleansing.

Relax before and after eating to help digestion.

Learn about herb teas. Add some to your diet.

Drink spring water instead of tap water unless you know that the area's water is pollutant-free.

Put on your plate only the amount you feel you can eat.

Try to add a couple of teaspoons of bran daily to your diet. Bran is the outer layer of the wheat kernel that is removed by modern day milling. It also is one of the best sources of fiber (bulk), which the intestines and colon so vitally need.

Eat cottage cheese. It's high in protein.

Seeds (sunflower, pumpkin, etc.) are high in nutritive value. They are delicious as toppings on salads, cereals, and desserts and wonderful as snacks.

Eat yogurt and kefir; they contain the bacteria needed for intestines.

Eat fruits in season.

Eat and/or serve foods you dislike, but should eat, in a new way, or introduce them to your diet in smaller portions.

Grow and eat your own sprouts: alfalfa, mung bean, wheat grass, etc. They are living, nutritious, tasty, easy to grow—and cheap. To grow your own: In a one quart wide-mouth jar pour $1/4$ inch of beans or seeds (in a two quart wide-mouth jar pour $1/2$ inch of beans or seeds). The actual number will vary, of course, according to the different sizes of the seeds and beans. Pour in twice as much water. Let it sit overnight or 8–10 hours in a dark place. Rinse with cool water and continue to rinse three times a day for the next three days. Let your sprouts have a day in the light to get some chlorophyll before eating. To drain water, punch holes inside out in the lid or use a screen lid.

Food Supplements

Deciding on a diet that suits your individual needs is, for the most part, trial and observation. While on the path to the right varieties of foods for you, it might be necessary to take food supplements. It is best to get vitamins and minerals directly from your diet, but it is sometimes necessary to take supplements.

Recent discoveries by pharmacologists have made remarkable breakthroughs in mental illness, using vitamins to balance the bodymind.

Where do you start with the food supplements? There are so many vitamins, minerals, wheat germs, yeasts, etc. One way is to get a blood and urine analysis. That will give you a pretty good idea of what your deficiencies are.

Chapter 15

Other Ways of Healing

The subject of modern Western medicine and its treatment of disease is the center of much controversy these days. The health of this country has too long been treated as the private preserve of the medical industry. It is time we become aware of what individuals themselves can do to maintain health and prevent illness. To prevent dis-ease before it starts is the goal.

In America today we tend to look at modern Western medicine as the only valid healer. Other systems of healing are often seen as primitive, faddish, ineffective, antiquated, mystical, or just plain nonsense. While one cannot deny the outstanding achievements of modern medicine, especially in the control and management of infectious diseases and the development of technical surgical procedures, let us not lose sight of the fact that the oldest and wisest healer known to man is the body-mind itself. It has been through an impressive evolution. The most any healing system can do is get the bodymind prepared to do its own work.

Bernard Jensen, M.D., a well-known author and lecturer on health and healing, believes that "The true healing art is one in which we teach a patient to change his living habits to conform to natural laws so that, instead of having to rebuild a sick body, he can prevent disease in the first place." This section is concerned with preventing dis-ease as well as finding corrective procedures. You will learn some of these diagnoses and preventative and healing techniques, both ancient and new. Some of the techniques, however, may seem far-fetched and harsh—but they are here to strengthen your natural powers of resistance. They may not correct every illness (when a body reaches the complaining stage, it's a more difficult time to start taking care of the ailment), but they won't do any harm. For the most part, they are very effective and work most of the time. Remember that nature needs time. The cure comes from within. Illness can be looked upon as a growth process—a sign to improve your health. Change your habits and stop dis-ease.

Kriyas

In yoga, cleansing processes known as Kriyas (the Sanskrit for "actions") are practiced to eliminate poisons from the body. These kriyas are used in ashrams and yoga hospitals as preventive and curative methods. The actions are designed to cleanse and stimulate parts of the internal body. You will recognize some of them, for they have been incorporated into Western therapies. They may be a "bit hard to handle" when you first hear about them—but they do the job. These should not be done without consulting your physician.

Nasal Cleansing

Removes dust, dirt, accumulated mucus; stimulates sinuses, eyes, ears; and prevents sinus headaches, asthma, and snoring.

First, cup your palm so water can collect in your hand from the tap, lake, or stream. Add a pinch of salt ($\frac{1}{2}$ teaspoon to 1 cup of water). With mouth open, bend over while lifting water to right nostril. Inhale water forcibly, snuffing into right nostril, then immediately forcibly exhale, snorting out the water. Do the same with the left nostril. Lukewarm water is best.

This technique can be done several times until nostrils are breathing freely.

Gagging

Removes mucus from throat; awakens body; opens and relaxes throat and face muscles.

Place your finger far enough down your throat to make you gag but not retch. At the same time make a gagging or a coughing sound. You will invariably bring up an accumulation of mucus.

Do this in the morning before brushing your teeth.

Enemas

Constipation is a most common ailment in civilized societies. As a result of chronic constipation the colon—the garbage can of the body—becomes a cesspool of backed-up excrement and poisons. Hardened residues stick to the lining of the colon, filling up the little pockets. This causes a slow poisoning of the body. It is essential that the normal eliminative process be carried out in order to expel the poisons and help the colon work efficiently. Enemas can help this restoration. Cleansing of the colon helps cure constipation and causes elimination during a fast. Proceed by this method:

While on your knees, head near floor, insert enema nozzle into anus. Take as much water as comfortable (a pint to one quart of warm water with a squirt of lemon juice added). Contract anal sphincter muscle, holding water in up to one minute. Then release water into toilet.

Enemas are not meant to take the place of natural bowel movements.

Three other Kriyas—Stomach Pump, Forward Stretch, and Breath of Fire—are part of the regular E/W program.

Reflexology

Reflexology is the study and practice of massaging certain parts of the hands and feet in order to cause a reflex action or stimulation in another part of the body. Reflexologists claim feet are maps to internal organs and parts of the anatomy.

When pressure is applied to a certain point on the bottom of your foot, it sends some sort of impulse to the corresponding part of the body by nerve pathways to relax or stimulate, depending upon the needs of the overactive or sluggish organ. Some of these pathways have yet to be neurologically discovered; but *Gray's Anatomy* says that "many of the details concerning the paths taken by the fibers are still unknown, and we must rely heavily upon information obtained from animal experimentation, although it may not have been confirmed by clinical observations with human patients." It appears that, in the end of the pathway (some say it's not the end, but a sharp turn like a drain pipe), crystalline toxins are collected, indicating an acute or chronic problem at the other end. The crystals are often sharp and jagged and give a needlelike pain when pressed. Reflexologists think they are either carbonic or uric acid deposits.

The entire bottom of the foot should be massaged, with special attention to tender and sensitive areas. One drawback of foot reflexology is that it may hurt while you massage the tender places. The reflex points on the map are not exactly on target for every foot. Different people have different feet—and there is still some argument as to the placement of some organs. So you don't treat disorders by literally pinpointing massage, but by exploring an entire area, as seen on the chart (page 197).

Start the massage with the toes—the territory for the head—and work your way down the body. Give each toe a twist and gentle pull. Use mainly the front and side of your thumb to press into toes and feet in a small circular movement. Use a knuckle to get deeper when necessary. That's usually when you're over a calloused pad in the "body" of the foot. You will develop a sensitivity and be able to know when you are causing pain by pressing against a bone or when you are in contact with a crystal.

When massaging someone else, a crystal will feel gritty, like a piece of sand. Watch the person's face—sometimes the lightest touch can send a person off their seat; sometime you can see only a trace of discomfort in the face. Working with sensitivity, increase the pressure of the massage on the point of soreness to break up the crystal. The bloodstream will cleanse away the toxins.

Because we keep our feet enclosed in shoes, the muscles don't get the proper amount of exercise. It is said that primitive man did not suffer from many of civilization's ailments simply because he did not wear shoes or his footwear had soft, supple soles, thus receiving constant stimulation from the ground.

Don't let the simplicity of this method stop you from at least trying the massage a few times. Corrective results are not seen with all cases, but one thing is for sure—whether you give or receive a foot massage, it has a soothing and relaxing effect on a part of the body that definitely lacks attention.

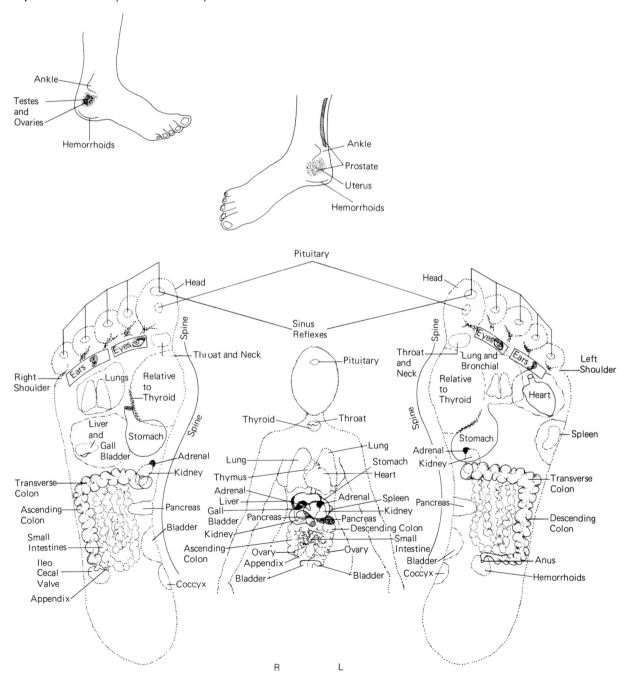

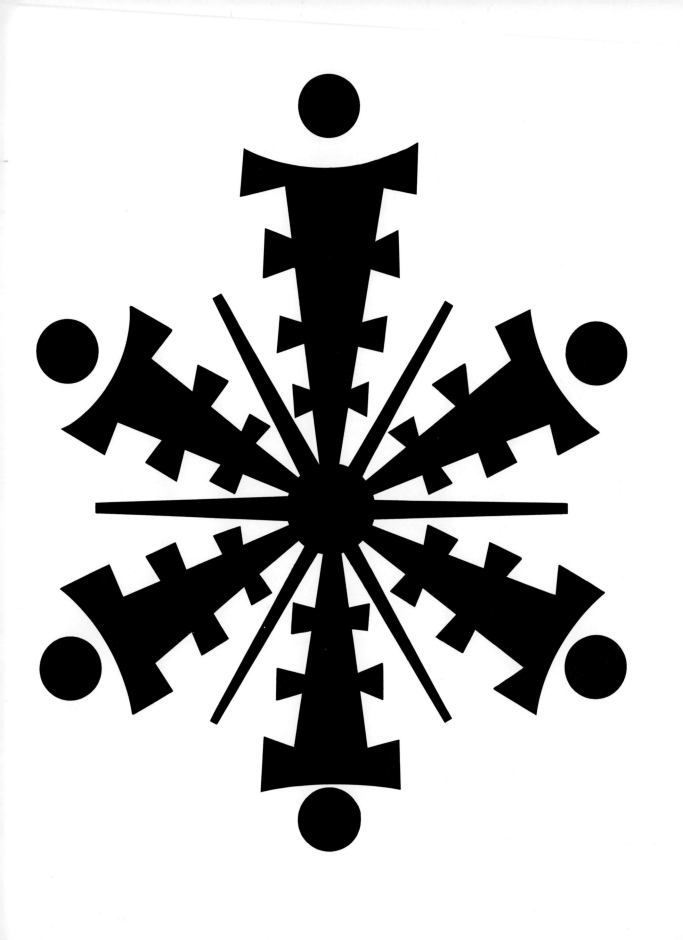

Tibetan Eye Chart

For generations the people of Tibet have used natural methods to correct visual weaknesses and improve their eyesight. Chief among the methods employed has been the use of certain exercises which have proved useful over long periods of time. The figure on this chart (page 198) was designed by Tibetan lama monks to give the necessary corrective exercises and stimulation to the muscles and nerves of the optical system. A few minutes of daily practice morning and evening will produce immediate effects, and, if maintained over a period of months, will effect definite improvement.

Eye Exercises

The eyes are influenced by the condition of the muscles that hold them in place. A great many eyesight disorders come from strain and tension. Add to this strain the hours we spend in front of the TV, at work under artificial lights and in the flickering entertainment of the movies.

One key to better vision is bodymind and eye relaxation. In addition to the eye exercises in the E/W program, here are some to relax and strengthen your eyes. These eye exercises can be used by everyone.

How to Use the Chart

Place the chart on a wall with the center spot in line with the nose when the head is held level. Standing erect and close to the wall, touch the tip of nose to the center spot on the chart. With head still, move the eyes clockwise around the outer edges (second tier from center for first few weeks) of each arm of the figure, including the black spots, until the starting point is reached. Repeat the movement in a counterclockwise direction. Blink and relax the eyes after each cycle; then do a half minute of palming (place the palms of each hand over each eye). Repeat as desired—but be careful to avoid strain.

Palming

Palming helps relax eyes and reduces eyestrain. Here's how to do it.

1 In a comfortable position close eyes lightly and place a cupped palm over each eye.
2 If you experience anything but pure black your bodymind and eyes are not relaxed. You may experience shades, shapes, textures of blackness, colors.
3 Center on a beautiful, joyful, serene setting where you like to be. Breathe long and deep.

4   Use your imagination to experience pure blackness. Do not strain to find it.

When you experience pure blackness without shades or shadows, your eyes are relaxed. Rest in this place. Do palming for from 5 to 10 minutes up to an hour. If you lie in the Corpse Pose, get a couple of pillows to prop up your elbows and arms so they don't strain. It's the total bodymind relaxation we are after. Remember the hands contain thousands of little nerve centers that exert a healing effect.

Fasting

Fasting is the abstention partially or totally from food and/or drink over a period of time, from hours to months (sometimes called a monodiet). Fasting has been used, to one degree or another, for many purposes throughout history—as a mental discipline, as a religious ritual, and as a type of therapeutic healing.

No doubt our ancestors first fasted when they noticed that animals stop eating when they are sick. Today many of us do just the opposite when we are ill. We feed the illness. Our intelligent body is already working overtime to eliminate the disease and we make things worse by eating a healthy meal to "give us energy." Actually, this just adds an extra amount of work for the body, causing it to send blood to the stomach and intestine to aid digestion.

You don't need to feel ill to benefit from fasting. Fasting is like spring cleaning for the body. During a fast the body burns and decomposes accumulations of fat, dead tissue, body toxins, mucus, pesticides, drugs, chemicals, and diseased tissue. During this time there is an increased elimination of poisons, which pass out through the urine (which is dark), skin (as eruptions), lungs and tongue (as foul breath), and bowel movements. It is during this period that some people experience a "healing crisis." It could be as mild as a headache or as bad as a fever—feeling worse than when you started. This is the inner doctor at work eliminating poisons.

Remember that these effects sometimes can be serious, and there is a large body of medical authority opposed to fasting. Always consult your physician before and during a fast to insure proper supervision, especially if you are suffering from serious illness or disease.

While fasting on juices and raw fruits the poisons are released slowly and are diluted so the body can eliminate them safely. Enemas help eliminate the poisons and taking Vitamin C helps neutralize them. Fasting rests and cleanses the intestinal tract, liver, and blood. A distended stomach will shrink and tend to resume its normal size. It is said that cholesterol will loosen and melt away.

You do not have to lie in bed to fast. In fact, many people have an abundance of energy during the fast. However, you may become tired during prolonged fasting. Your bodymind will be the best indicator. Remember: it takes will power to stay on a fast, especially the first few times when people tell you how bad and tired you will feel.

Begin with a twenty-four-hour fast; eat as much as you want of one fruit or one vegetable. Gradually you can build to extend the fast and lower consumption. Several one-day fasts are a good beginning to cleansing your system. They will also give you the confidence and experience to graduate to the longer fasts. Ten days should be the longest fast without expert supervision.

Suggested Fasts

Here is a detoxifying diet: mix 2 tablespoons of lemon juice and 2 tablespoons of blackstrap molasses with 8 ounces of medium-hot water. Drink from six to twelve glasses a day. Use pure maple syrup or sorghum as alternatives to the molasses. (I recommend the pure maple syrup.) The drink tastes like hot lemonade. It is suggested that you remain on this diet up to ten days—for the beginning faster, however, only a few days is suggested. The eleventh morning, or the day after the one you have decided to be your last day, change to orange juice mixed with water. That night eat a bowl of fresh vegetable soup and rye crackers. On the twelfth day, continue orange juice in the morning; add vegetable soup at lunch and vegetable salad for dinner. On the thirteenth day, drink orange juice and eat small portions of brown rice and vegetables. On the fourteenth day you can resume normal food intake. This diet should not be used by those with hypoglycemia or diabetes.

If you have any chronic problems, show this fast to a doctor before you begin. Fasts over seven days in polluted cities are not advised. Once you start fasting, you will find there are all kinds of fasts, diets, and combinations, using, for example, fruits in season. One you'll find hard to beat is carrot juice (with a bit of celery or beet). It pays to have a juicer for this one, but you can buy the juice in bottles or, better yet, get it fresh at a juice bar. The list of vitamins carrot juice contains and what it cures needs a chapter itself. Up to five days is a good period for a carrot juice fast. You can chew a few carrots a day to obtain bulk to aid the peristalsis needed to remove toxins.

Many times during a fast you become constipated. There may not be enough bulk in the colon to get the peristalsis working properly. Of course, you should never take drugs to remedy this. There are several techniques you can choose. One technique already mentioned is an enema. Herbal teas can also do the trick. A colonic enema is usually administered by a naturopathic doctor. A fourth method is recommended by Stanley Burroughs: in the morning before eating or drinking juice, drink 1 quart of warm water with a tablespoon of sea salt added. I recommend you give yourself at least an hour and a half close to a toilet. It works well. (This technique is rather drastic. It eliminates large quantities of water, is distasteful, and sometimes causes temporary abdominal pains.)

Working with these different techniques, you can choose the one best and most comfortable for you.

Breaking a fast the right way is as important as starting one. The transition back to normal eating should be done slowly. The length of the fast, of course, determines the transition period back to normal food intake. Break a twenty-four-hour fast with a raw vegetable salad, using lemon juice as a dressing. The salad can be followed by one or two steamed vegetables. Do not break a fast with animal products—i.e., cheese, milk, meat, fish—or with nuts or seeds. However, your second meal after a one-day fast can include light amounts of these products. Breaking a two-to-eight-day fast or mono diet (eating one food), you return to normal eating more slowly. Stay away from heavy foods. Eat lightly of foods that contain water, like fruits and vegetables. Popcorn acts as a good broom, sweeping out your digestive tract. A ten-day fast needs three days as a transition period, as previously mentioned. The main thing to remember is to chew the food well, eat slowly, and do not overeat.

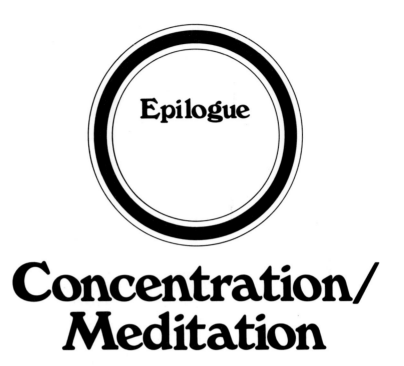

Concentration/ Meditation

Concentration

". . . Concentration, which is necessary prelude to Meditation, aims at unwavering focus on a chosen thing or idea to the exclusion of any other . . . [it is] complete one-pointedness of thought upon the subject in hand, be it a pencil, a virtue, or a diagram imagined in the mind," says Christmas Humphreys in *Concentration and Meditation.*

Some techniques teach concentration before meditation. Concentration is the process of fixing the mind on an object—external or internal—to focus the energy of attention. In a normal waking state of consciousness, attention is scattered, thoughts are dispersed, constantly draining energy from the bodymind. You feel it after a day of constant mental bombardment. Mind chatter sabotages concentration. Concentration techniques work on stopping the mind chatter.

If concentration is fixing or focusing on one point, meditation is the art of going from one-pointedness to no-point—being the whole—and going from a little self into a greater Self.

Meditation

"We are not in quest of holiness but of youth—the eternal youth of a being who grows" (Satprem, disciple of Sri Aurobindo).

Meditation is a natural outgrowth and compliment to the E/W exercise program. E/W exercise works on the body—meditation on the mind. Remember the body and mind are two complementary and interdependent aspects of the whole being. We can't totally change the physical habits without changing the psychological habits—and vice versa. It takes total effort.

The medical uses of meditation should be mentioned here. Studies using biofeedback apparatus have confirmed the amazing physiological control Zen and yogi meditation masters have over involuntary systems—heart rate, blood pressure, and body temperature. What seems more important is that even nonmeditators show a degree of control when tested. Evidence from biofeedback studies also shows that meditation reduces high blood pressure, hypertension, headaches, migraines, digestive disorders, insomnia, stress, fatigue, and nervousness.

Meditation is a growth process of expanding consciousness. There is an undoing of conditioning—compulsive and habitual behavior of the bodymind. Meditation resolves whatever has made one's awareness narrow and shallow in the first place.

The aim is not to take you away into some deep trance, but to bring you closer in harmony with the world around you.

Probably one of the most well-known forms is Transcendental Meditation. The term transcendental means "going beyond." The founder of TM, Maharishi Mahesh Yogi, says TM gives a meditator his own *mantra* (the Sanskrit word for "hymn" or "phrase") to work with. Transcendental Meditation has had a great deal of success in the Western world. It is easily learned and has immediate effects without absorbing the meditator in any religious doctrine or way of life. All that is necessary is to sit and recite silently your own mantra, as prescribed by one of Maharishi's teachers for 20–30 minutes twice daily. Maharishi claims TM puts you in touch with the creative intelligence that lies deep in the recesses of one's own psyche. This allows one to realize one's unique potential.

In addition to Transcendental Meditation, there are many other forms of meditation which use techniques such as repeating a word or a phrase silently in any language. Herbert Benson, a research psychologist at Harvard, gets relaxation results similar to Transcendental Meditation in his lab, using the word "one." Ramana Maharishi, an Indian Saint, used a simple self inquiry "who am I?" The *rinzai* school of Zen employs the use of a riddlelike question called a *koan*—"What is the sound of one hand clapping?" There is no particular answer, but the student uses the question to focus attention.

Another technique—with the eyes open—is when the meditator centers his attention on a picture, symbol, statue, or candle flame. Attention can also be focused on the rhythm of the breath or some point on/in the body, such as the third eye (a point an inch above the brows), the heart, or the Hara (just below the navel). Some forms of meditation combine movement, as do Sufi whirling dervishes, Zen techniques of walking, and T'ai Chi and other martial arts. Biofeedback instruments can also be an aid to meditation.

In most of the different forms there is an attitude to keep in mind—be free from any goal for the meditation. As Baba Ramdas says, "Desires and motives affect perception."

Take one minute right now. Sit comfortably in an easy pose or on a chair, close your eyes, and still the mind. Every distraction leads away from a still mind. Every thought, meaningful or meaningless, takes you away from being here now. In watching you begin to see the movement of your thoughts. Some teachers will say that those thoughts are not a disturbance, but an object of meditation, not to be suppressed, but looked upon with awareness and comprehension.

Meditation produces a solid feeling of oneself, a presence, poise, balance, and inner harmony to excel in life's game of living and loving. A master in meditation, Claudio Naranjo, says in *Psychology of Meditation*, "This presence or mode of being transforms whatever it touches. If its medium is movement, it will turn into dance; if stillness, into living sculpture; if thinking, into the higher reaches of intuition; if sensing, into a merging with the miracle of being; if feeling, into love; if singing, into sacred utterance; if speaking, into prayer or poetry; if doing the things of ordinary life, into a ritual in the name of God or a celebration of existence."

If you want to know what meditation is you must experience it directly. The place of meditation is especially important at first. You can use the same place you exercise, but it must be free of harsh noise. A quiet spot in the country is wonderful, but not always accessible. Here are a few concentration/meditation techniques to get you started.

The lotus posture is the one in which we see Buddha sitting (left foot on right thigh, right foot on left thigh). It is considered by ancient and modern masters the most useful for purposes of meditation. Many people can not sit in the lotus; if you can't, then sit cross-legged in Easy Pose. You can even sit on a chair with your feet on the floor. In any case, put a pillow or cushion under your buttocks, keep your back straight, and breathe slow and easy.

Attend to the Breath
Close your eyes (later you can try it with your eyes open) and be aware of your breathing. Be aware of your abdomen moving in and out. Feel the air rush in and out through your nose. Feel your physical body relax on every exhalation. Imagine the layers of muscle tension peeling back, letting oxygen into the cells to rejuvenate them. Count each exhalation until ten. Then start over. Thoughts will enter—watch them and let them go—get back to the counting and watching the breath. Do not try to push thoughts out of your mind—they will only intensify—back to the object of attention. This is not a breathing exercise.

Falling asleep may be a problem at first, but it will pass—that's all in the growth process.

Mantra
In the sitting position, repeat the Tibetan phrase *Om mani padme hum* silently to yourself, over and over. When thoughts rush into your mind replace them with the phrase. *Om* (sum total of all energy) *mani* (jewel or crystal) *padme* (lotus) *hum*

(heart)—or, as Baba Ramdas says, "The entire universe is just like a pure jewel or crystal right in the heart or center of the lotus flower, which is me." In esoteric language, the Path inward is a jeweled path. Superconsciousness is more often associated with brilliant illumination and flashing colors. The qualities of inner world have a permanence like the brilliance of the colors emitted from precious stones.

Words and their rhythms set up vibrations that effect the bodymind. Ramdas says, "The conscious beings who evolve certain languages, such as Sanskrit, specifically evolve the sounds of these languages to be connected with various states of consciousness—unlike the English language—so that a Sanskrit mantra, if you do it over and over again, will take you to a certain state of consciousness." Raise your vibrations—and lower your tension.

Om can be used alone as a mantra. It is said to include all the sounds in the universe. *Om* is pronounced *aum*. A starts in the back of the throat. *U* rolls over the roof of the mouth into the *m*, lightly tingling on gently closed lips. *Om* sounds like "home." First repeat it softly aloud, then internalize the sound.

I am healthy now is another phrase that can be repeated. In fact, you can change *healthy* to any positive word you choose.

The Witness
This is a place where you watch your thoughts while sitting and actions while doing. You will see how the thoughts come into view and how they leave without becoming involved yourself. You can practice this while sitting and then carry it over into everyday living. When you see the chattering thought—and see it is getting in your way—simply say *stop*. This place of the witness is used as a technique in the growth process, not a dissociation out of anxiety.

The Flame
Controlled gaze, focusing on an external object, will also quiet the mind. Concentrate on a candle a few feet in front of you while in the sitting position. It is all right to blink your eyes; they may water. If your eyes begin to strain, close them and do palming until refreshed. Then continue concentration. When thoughts enter the mind, bring the candle back into focus.

Start with ten to twenty minutes of these techniques once a day. Try to do them the same time each day. It takes time to quiet a mind that's been on the loose for a lifetime. Don't be discouraged. When the mind is calmed you will be able to see more clearly without looking through the individual prejudices which affect your perception and inhibit your growth.

No one technique is right for everyone. It's left open for you to find your own meditative path. Any technique that works for you is a good one. You will find your own way of integration. The ultimate meditation has no technique. It comes from the sound of the surf breaking on a beach or the sight of a flight of geese in formation over a lovely landscape. Naranjo says, "theoretically, any meditation object could suffice and be equivalent to any other, particular objects of meditation serve (especially for one not far advanced in the practice) the double function of a target of attention and a reminder of that right attitude which is both the path and the goal of meditation."